COVID –

A FRONTLINE DOCTOR'S VIEW

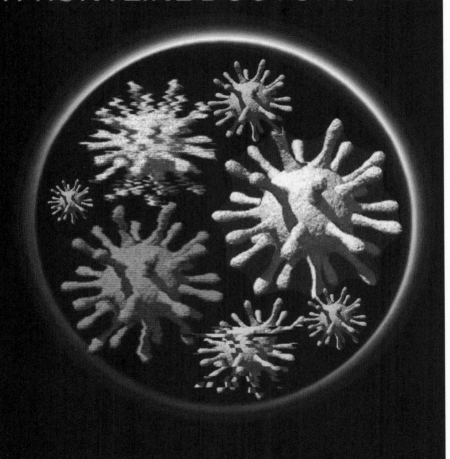

CAXTON OPERE, MD

Other Books by the Author

The HCQ Debate: What Did Researchers Hide
Covid-19: Physician Treatment Strategies.
Divorce Medicine: How Divorce and Toxic Relationships Affect Your Health.
Female Sexual Arousal and The Pink Pill
25 Things Every Pastor Must L.I.K.E. About Divorce
Covid-19 Remedies
GSP: God's Success Program

COVID-19: REMEDIES

A Frontline Doctor's View

Caxton Opere, MD

COVID-19 REMEDIES: A Frontline Doctor's View

ISBN: 978-1-952642-00-5
Published by Divorce Prevention Inc.
Frisco, TX, USA

DISCLAIMER

TABLE OF CONTENTS

Never trust anyone that tells you after you've been diagnosed with Covid-19, to go home, fold your arms and just wait.
-    Caxton Opere, MD

ACKNOWLEDGEMENTS

To my two late Grandmothers, for introducing me to remedies that work, even though I didn't believe in them as an internist until the pandemic came and we were told not to prescribe any drugs for early treatment of Covid-19,

To my wife and children. Thank you. This book would never have been written without your love and unwavering support,

To the individuals and families that lost loved ones to Covid-19,

To the first responders nurses and healthcare workers who died following exposure in the line of Covid-19 duty,

To those doctors and nurses who continue to work relentlessly to find a solution if not a cure to covid-19, treating patients and standing up to the impending tyranny,

To the others around the world like Steve Kirsch, who put up millions of dollars of their own money for clinical trials to find effective treatments for Covid-19,

To those involved in non-skewed medical reporting about Covid-19 and investigate and exposing the truth and to the absolute truth seekers who are not interested in a one-sided narrative,

Lastly to you the reader, for without you, all the information in this book would never be seen, heard, understood or applied.

Thank you.

Tribute to Frontline Covid-19 Workers:

Special Tribute to Hospital Staff, (Tribute from 1st edition)

We cannot thank the frontline workers enough. You might think that means only doctors and nurses as well as lab techs and respiratory therapists. My biggest thanks is to the house-keeping staff of all the facilities around the world that continue to provide their services to make our healthcare facilities decent, sanitary, professional environments we are proud of. Even though overcrowded at this pandemic period, hospitals still represent the best places to work and give most of us a sense of pride and joy. I've always held a lot of respect for this humble group, the housekeeping team. They give every hospital its aura of neatness, style and completeness.

As a physician for over thirty-one years and board certified in internal medicine, I have always enjoyed patient care and working on the frontlines. I don't know the details of the frustrations other healthcare professionals face today, but I have firsthand knowledge of the pain many physicians experience as they practice medicine in 2021.

Many doctors have been forced into unnecessary, unproductive, unrealistic work pathways that hinder the flow and expression of their abilities and effectiveness, autonomy and perhaps even talents. The very reason many chose this profession has been snatched out of their hands and the sense of accomplishment and autonomy that previously accompanied the end of a doctor's workday has been turned into a sigh as they manage to get out of the hospital. More than 50% of physicians in my calling as an emergency medicine physician and internist are burnt out. At a time when the brilliant minds in medicine should be meeting to figure out a treatment combination that would work against Covid-19, doctors may find themselves without personal protective equipment and threats from some hospital administrators. It's almost as if there is a doctor envy from those engaged in administrative tasks in such hospitals. Our creativity is stalled, our personalities stifled, our autonomy strangled and our endurance stretched beyond what is socially, physiologically, and mentally permissible. All this is reflected in the current burnout rates of US physicians and then suddenly, Covid-19 strikes. Only doctors can strike back. If hospitals don't listen to their doctors, but instead hire ignorant or medically illiterate people to create electronic health records, wield administrative wands of authority threateningly over healthcare providers for suggesting better pathways of care or workflow, the end may be closer than we think. Doctors are being threatened or fired for speaking up regarding personal protective equipment! It's no longer news. Many doctors work under very poor conditions in the US despite the massive resources available. Stick a Q-tip into the air-conditioning in some doctor's call rooms and lounges and you'll be shocked we're still breathing. Look at the keyboards of computers in the doctor's lounge or workrooms in the hospital and you'll get a better idea yourself. While many hospitals have excellent facilities and administrators that care about physicians, particularly their hospitalists, all a physician has to do sometimes, is to pick the wrong place to work, agree to the wrong sets of conditions when signing a contract, and their life becomes a living hell. The fight for the truth in providing the best care to our patients must not be ignored.

Kudos to all the amazing doctors, nurses, physician extenders, nurses, respiratory therapists on the planet, especially those battling with Covid-19 on the frontlines. God bless you and protect you all.

"If we lose our doctors and nurses to illness, we have no line of defense to fight this disease, as access to healthcare services will diminish rapidly".
- Patrice Harris, MD. AMA President 2020

Preface to the First Edition

This book as well as its companion for physicians, *Covid-19: Physician Treatment Strategies* were written as an urgent response to assist in the fight against the Covid-19 pandemic. It is what in the business world is called a minimum viable product and is not written to attest to any academic or clinical superiority but to address a pandemic that could potentially decimate millions if left unchecked. As a frontline emergency medicine and hospital medicine physician, I know there is great value in having firsthand knowledge of what is in this book. The information here should go beyond the pandemic period, lower the overuse of healthcare services, and, reduce time off from work due to other incurable but mild viral illnesses and colds. If you're infected with Covid-19 or suspect you have been exposed, call your doctor and follow your local health authority's recommendations and instructions. Reading this book does not negate any recommendations mandated by drug manufacturers, professional societies or authoritative clinical guidelines.

It seems that with the information gathered from the frontlines that Covid-19 attacks the entire body systems in such a virulent manner that if we fold our arms and wait till a vaccine is developed, too many will die. I have written this treatise because it now seems obvious that everyone involved directly or indirectly with the care of Covid-19 patients needs to start thinking of a cure or treatment strategy and do so outside the box. That's because even a 5 to 7 month period for developing a vaccine as opposed to the typical ten-year period for developing such vaccines is now too long. If nothing is done, many lives will be lost prematurely, unnecessarily and negligently.

The book describes remedies that should be easily available, affordable and over the counter as well as incontrovertible therapies that informed doctors and other practitioners should never be afraid to prescribe or recommend to you when requested.

Prior to the pandemic, most practicing physicians were unfamiliar with the important role of nutritional supplements in boosting the immune system. We downplayed its importance in protecting against viral infections. We have finally come to terms with their effectiveness in this role and most doctors now take their vitamins regularly. Many of us routinely mocked patients that presented with viral or mild bacterial infections if they told us they would take the remedies prescribed in this book. Many got better with their own self-administered remedies but healthcare professionals including myself thought they had some lose mental screws. That has changed, a legacy left by this pandemic! The world will always be a better place because of it.

April 7, 2020.

Preface to the Second Edition

Denying early treatment in Covid-19 and taking a firm stand against such treatment is ignorance at best. Many Covid-19 deaths resulted not just from the infection but from the lack of knowledge in the medical community on early treatment strategies besides wearing masks and social distancing. This lack of information was my major reason for writing the first edition of this book as well as the physician's version, *COVID-19: Physician Treatment Strategies*, still available on www.smashword.com and other online stores. After *Covid-19 Remedies* was submitted for publishing and blocked by Amazon on April 8, 2020, the misinformation from government agencies, the mainstream media, by those with a vaccine-only agenda escalated. In addition, news of Covid-19 recoveries were downplayed by the media, while direct attacks on doctors proposing or showing the value of early treatment strategies continued. As a result, we have over 3 million dead globally from Covid-19 as of June 12, 2021. Another 176 million people are infected worldwide. That's more than double the combined population of Iran, Turkey or any European country. Those who survived have lost jobs, and loved ones, while some are now chronic haulers of Covid-19. Too many have been negatively impacted on a global scale by the un-curtailed infection, deaths, and ravaging economic losses. While emergency department visits had dropped by 24% in the United States and by 88% in Argentina, the May-October 2020 issue of Canada's *Public Health Ontario Rapid Review* reported increased mental health visits, increased severity of illness at presentation due to delayed care. Adolescent anxiety, alcohol use and suicidal thoughts have all risen. We can do something to change this pathetic condition. Together.
June 24, 2021

Introduction

At the onset of the pandemic, I was concerned that the authorities in the United States were not providing useful treatment information about Covid-19 to healthcare professionals. They seemed more concerned about telling us "what not to prescribe. Thank God for outliers such as Drs. Didier Raoult, Stella Emmanuel, Simone Gold, Paul Marik, Pierre Kory and others, including the "mysterious coroner" who saved an entire city from Covid-19 by prescribing early treatment. Without the "no treatment" propaganda, fewer will have died.

Outside the United States, many doctors have been prescribing early drug treatments for Covid-19 patients successfully. Many of these non-US doctors and practitioners are also recommending vaccinations for Covid-19 patients. With the exception of Canada and Australia of course! In the US, the doctors have been split. We have doctors who do not see the role of any agent in early treatment for Covid-19. They maintain their position by citing tainted scientific data, naively believing science cannot be used to tell a lie. Some of these doctors also launch attacks on doctors that have critically sifted through the data and have decided to treat early Covid-19 patients with pre-approved drugs. If you don't get an opportunity to be treated early for Covid-19 by such doctors, you may find this book very helpful.

Unfortunately, doctors that cannot see the value of early treatments have always posed a real danger to the wellbeing of those seeking such early treatments from them. Unable to critically assess the literature yet priding themselves on analysis obtained from news outlet doctors that may have been paid by vaccine manufacturers, these doctors refuse to treat patients and watch them die or get seriously ill and hospitalized, following infection with Covid-19. This group of uninformed or rather ill-informed doctors is one reason the pandemic is still with us.

I recently listened to a Clubhouse® room conversation where seven doctors attacked a fellow doctor. The latter said he had successfully treated thirty patients for Covid-19 with drugs. The treating doctor thought he was sharing useful information. These seven doctors, one of them a cardiologist, descended on the treating doctor like a vulture and ripped him apart. The others joined in. It was only about the data and the methodology. None of them bothered to ask this doctor how his patients presented, if they had a fever, low oxygen levels, their ages, vital signs, duration of symptoms, comorbidities, or their overall clinical condition. None of them was curious enough to find out what he treated his patients with, or the dosages, for how long, or how long it took the patients to recover. In effect, they never asked any of the important clinical questions any good doctor would want to know about a sick set of Covid-19 patients, even if the methodology was wrong. All they cared about was the data. They didn't know that the father of evidence based medicine, the late Professor David Sackett and three other brilliant professors of medicine defined evidence-based medicine not just solely as a data-driven practice, but as:

> "the **conscientious** explicit and **judicious** use of current best evidence in making decisions about the **care** of **individual patients**. (Sackett, DL., Haynes, RB., Guyatt, GH & P., Tugwell. Clinical Epidemiology: A Basic Science for Clinical Medicine. 1991)

The key words in bold letters are **conscientious**, **judicious** and **care** of **individual patients**. Doctors can gather all the best evidence, but until they know how to care for individual patients judiciously and in all good conscience using the best evidence, all they've gathered, is in vain. Sadly these "magnificent seven" doctors demonstrated to the public that they lacked a good conscience and were only interested in their data, not in the condition of the patients treated. What they did to the treating doctor was dehumanizing and it got me wondering how little compassion is left in the medical profession. I had an opportunity to speak to this vilified doctor a few days later. To my surprise, he not only admitted to having received his mRNA vaccine shots, he would not deprive patients of vaccines they needed in his practice. His only crime was that he provided early treatment for Covid-19 patients. The "panel of seven" obviously got it wrong when they presumed that by providing early treatment to Covid-19 patients, this doctor was anti-vaccine or anti-Covid-19 mRNA vaccine. Today, I spoke with another Covid-19 post-vaccination long-hauler female. The same group of doctors had harassed her. From what they did, a lawsuit might be pending on them as they took a picture of her profile and posted it on social media platforms requesting she be banned. Such bedside manners! I would therefore not recommend you go around a group of doctors who may lack the moral and ethical mindset of a truly scientifically open-minded approach and expect them to respect your perspective on the new vaccines or your pain after getting complications from the jabs.

When one listener asked the seven doctors what they would do if they saw a patient with early Covid-19, one of them said they would just treat it like the "common cold". Unbelievable! Imagine a doctor calling Covid-19 "like the common cold" in June 2021! The doctor went mute when another listener challenged him to such folly. It was obvious that while these doctors had data-driven strategies, they did not have a clinically driven approach to caring for Covid-19 patients based on the currently available evidence. They were at best scientists, but not doctors in the real world sense of it. Many of these "doctors" are probably unaware that *randomized control trials* could also become *randomized control tricks*. You should read *The HCQ Debate: What Did Researchers Hide* to learn more about these tricks!

Outside the United States, pro-vaccine doctors are recommending vaccines and providing early Covid-19 treatment using pre-approved drugs. In the real world of patient care, the two, that is, vaccines and early treatment of Covid-19 with drugs, should go hand in hand. So why is there so much animosity towards early treatment by pro-vaccine doctors and the powerful media in the United States? Why do journalists try to rip you apart as a doctor or politician if you were "caught" mentioning any effective treatments for Covid-19? And why were doctors expected to fold their arms, do nothing for their Covid-19 patients and simply wait eleven months for the vaccine to arrive? Why weren't US government officials leading the world in treatment strategies? The answer to these questions requires a review of the entire Covid-19 history. While this history is tainted by politics, the primary driver of Covid-19 seemed to be profit. How much profit is potentially involved here, and at what cost to human lives?

In the United States alone, there have been over 600,000 deaths from Covid-19! That's the population of 100 small US towns, or over two hundred times the number of people killed on September 11, 2001. Why did so many people have to die while waiting for a vaccine? Was there nothing that could have been used to treat Covid-19 patients while we waited for a vaccine? If there was, why were the authorities silent about it? Does the behavior of our government officials show that they care about the number of deaths, more than two hundred times deaths from 9/11? The answer to this question came in the form of a document released in January 2017 by the US Department of Health and Human Services (DHHS) and the Food and Drug Administration (FDA). That document explained the conditions for granting emergency use authorization (EUA) for any new drug or vaccine.

Let me simplify what happens before a new drug or vaccine is brought to your local pharmacy. Before a vaccine manufacturer releases their new vaccine to the public, it must first be rigorously tested in animals and then man. That is, you test animals, obtain all the necessary data on safety and efficacy in these, before introducing the drug or vaccine into humans. The usual progression is from mice, to monkeys and finally to humans. If the vaccine or drug passes the safety and efficacy requirements in the particular animal species, the pregnant females of that species are then tested as appropriate. If the researchers started with mice, pregnant mice should then be tested. Next in line will be monkeys. If the monkeys are tested successfully, then pregnant monkeys should be tested. Then depending on the outcomes of these animal studies, the drug can then be introduced into humans and subsequently into pregnant women and children.

There is often a regulatory arm of government that decides whether or not a vaccine or drug is acceptable for use in humans. In the United States, the Food and Drug Administration (FDA) performs this regulatory role. A pharmaceutical company files an Investigational New Drug Application (INDA form 1571) with the FDA. The company can start testing the new drug in clinical trials thirty days after sending in their INDA form; they do not need FDA "approval" before starting their clinical trials. This 30-day period allows the FDA to perform a brief evaluation and if necessary, place the INDA on hold. In most instances the new drug or biologic agent (vaccines, monoclonal antibodies) would have been tested as mentioned above for a few years before the INDA is filed. Once the drug or vaccine successfully undergoes phase III clinical trials, the sponsor, that is, the pharmaceutical company, files a New Drug Application (NDA) with the FDA (form FDA 356h). This must be filed before bringing a drug or vaccine to the marketplace. The FDA rates new chemical entities (NCEs) such as the Covid-19 mRNA vaccines as either type A, B or C, depending on the therapeutic potential offered by the new agent. The sponsor must also send in an annual report within 60 days of the anniversary of the approval of the NDA using form 2252. (Bert Spilker, 1991). If we see the drug at our local pharmacy, it means it passed all the stringent requirements in appropriate clinical trials.

The average pregnancy duration for mice is 21 days, monkeys 175 days, and humans 280 days.

Safety trials for a new drug or vaccine should evaluate pregnant females in any given species for a minimum of the duration of pregnancy in that species. While this step may be partially bypassed in unusual situations like life-threatening cancers or a decimating pandemic like Covid-19, genuine concern for the safety of babies and mothers cannot be overruled. The decision to give vaccines to reproductive age females, children and pregnant women must be based on a proper risk benefit analysis. You must know the risk of infection and risk of complications from the infection in untreated subjects in these groups. Absolute data about the safety of the vaccines must be made available. That means gathering data on severe complications from vaccinations. You should not give a vaccine to children or pregnant women in the general population without finding out the risk of getting Covid-19 in these specific groups. According to the CDC, most (90%) of severe allergic reactions (anaphylaxis) were in women.

According to Tom Shimabukuro, MD, MPH, MBA, deputy director of the CDC's Immunization Safety Office, there have been reports of myocarditis in 789 younger vaccine recipients 30 years and younger following vaccination with both the Pfizer-BioNTech and Moderna vaccines. This means researching the effects of the vaccine in a group of volunteer pregnant women, their offspring and in young children is now mandatory. If it is unethical to do such a study, then ethical and medical soundness of mass vaccination of women and children should be halted. For example, what if the baseline risk for severe Covid-19 in an unvaccinated child is far less than the risk of an adverse event from the vaccine itself? Rephrased, what if the risk of an adverse event from the vaccine is much higher than the risk of severe Covid-19 infection in an unvaccinated child? Should you still give that child the vaccine? Even though the incidence of Covid-19 in children is low, the incidence of adverse effects from the vaccine may be higher than expected benefit from giving the vaccine to low risk children.

The latest recommendation from the CDC dated April 21, 2021, is to continue vaccinating young children twelve years of age and older. There are several important unanswered questions regarding vaccination of children. First, what is the actual benefit-risk calculation in young children for these new mRNA vaccines specifically with respect to Covid-19? Do we have enough events in children to make such clinically relevant calculations? What is the likelihood of harm in children from the vaccine as a specific number? What is the likelihood of benefit as a specific number? What is the benefit-harm ratio? When did we as a people become so callous about children in the United States? The vaccines did not get sufficient animal studies to be approved for human use and should never be given to children except the benefit far outweighs the risk. I knew there was something wrong with the vaccines last year when Dr. Fauci started claiming the vaccine was "safe", just two months into the clinical trials. No one else in their right mind will tell you that a 2-month old vaccine is safe even if it has one hundred percent efficacy! To think America is supposed to be one of the safest places for a child in the entire world! Despite reports that people are dropping dead shortly after getting vaccinated, we not only ignore the statistics of the clinical trials, or adverse vaccine reports, we add insult to injury by recommending the vaccine to young children. Where are the evidence-based numbers on the risk benefit analysis that allows them to arrive at such a horrific conclusion to vaccinate children? While the myocarditis-pericarditis complication in children is short-term, the CDC is intentionally ignoring the potential long-term effects of these vaccines on growing children or the reproductive system of young females. I recently spoke with a doctor from India who said he had enrolled his two children in a clinical trial and sent me pictures! Some of his colleagues thought he was insane. He based his decision on a statistical term called relative risk reduction (RRR, Triple R). I have contended that the RRR is useful in highlighting tiny absolute differences between treated (vaccinated) and untreated (placebo) groups. When the absolute differences between the vaccinated group and the unvaccinated placebo groups are insignificant, statistics should not be reported in a way that misleads doctors and policy makers. If this deception is done by experienced professionals who have been studying and publishing scientific papers and statistically analyzing clinical trials, it should be considered a crime particularly as it relates to a pandemic. We will see how statistics has been misused in the next chapter.

Please read the disclaimer on page 4 of this book before you continue reading the rest of the book.

Chapter A!

Dangerously Manipulated Statistics!

You Don't Need A Course or Degree in Biostatistics!

One of the world's foremost leaders on clinical trials, Professor Bert Spilker, clearly stated in *A Guide To Clinical Trials, (Raven Press, New York. 1991)* that using relative risk reduction (RRR) to calculate the magnitude of a treatment does not adequately reflect the magnitude of the risk in those who did not receive the treatment. What Professor Spilker means is that when you use RRR, you may completely ignore or miss what happens in the untreated group and that what happened in this group may be far more important in obtaining the complete picture of how to use the results of the clinical trials.

As an illustration, let's say the results of a clinical trial have just been published in a prestigious medical journal. Only 4 people got sick in the vaccinated group while 80 people got sick in the placebo group. A layperson may quickly jump to the conclusion that the vaccine is twenty times better than the placebo. We may laugh at the layperson for jumping to such a conclusion, but should a statistics expert make the same mistake? The obvious answer is no! A statistically naïve person can fall into this RRR trap and arrive at the same conclusion as the naïve person. Calculating just the RRR will also give the impression that the vaccine is twenty times more effective at protecting people from illness than the placebo. It's not a direct inference but an implied one based on a simple calculation. Even if you don't like numbers or hate statistics, it's still quite easy to calculate the efficacy of the vaccine using the RRR formula.

Simply subtract the number of infected patients in the placebo group (80 patients) from the number of infected patients in the vaccinated group (4 patients). Then divide the result by the number of infected patients in the placebo group.

The calculations for vaccine efficacy will look like this:
> Number of infected patients in placebo group = 80
> Number of infected patients in placebo group = 4
> Vaccine Efficacy = RRR
> = (80-4)/80
> = (76/80) x 100%
> = 95%
> Vaccine efficacy is 95%.

A statistician therefore arrives at about the same conclusion regarding the vaccine's efficacy as the layperson. The only difference between them is that the statistician is using a slightly more sophisticated method, the relative risk reduction to arrive at the same conclusion.

This 95% efficacy for the vaccine doesn't change no matter what the total number of subjects in each group is. So assuming there are equal numbers of subjects in the vaccinated and placebo groups, it won't matter if there are 100, a million or one billion patients in each group. The vaccine efficacy will still be 95%. If you're pretty good with numbers you might immediately see that the absurdity of this calculation.

> If 80 out of ten thousand patients got infected in the placebo group, and 4 out of ten thousand got infected in the vaccinated group,
> The infection rate in the placebo group
> = 80 divided by 10,000
> = 0.008 x 100%
> = 0.8%

Again if 4 out of ten thousand patients got infected in the vaccinated group,
The infection rate in the vaccinated group
= 4 divided by 10,000
= 0.0004 x 100%
= 0.04%

Even if the infection rates in the placebo and vaccinated groups were 0.008% and 0.0004% respectively, or if the infection rates in the placebo and vaccinated groups were 0.00008% (80 of 100 million) and 0.000004% respectively (4 of 100 million), the vaccine efficacy will still be 95%. In the latter two instances the differences between the placebo and vaccinated group infection rates were 0.0076 and 0.000076% respectively! Insisting on vaccinating people because of the RRR-based vaccine efficacy must have another motive and bias driving such a decision and it's not a medical one. Whether it's 80 out of ten thousand or 80 out of ten billion people, the vaccine efficacy using RRR will always be 95% as long as the ratios between the vaccinated and unvaccinated subjects is kept the same at 80:4. So even if 99.99992% of the unvaccinated people do not get infected, the vaccine efficacy will still be 95%.

The real clinical problem is that the RRR doesn't tell you about the risk of infection in those who did not get the vaccine and that's what's not provided by the RRR vaccine efficacy calculation. This absurdity and redundancy is why Dr. Spilker's statement was introduced at the beginning of the chapter. No matter what you consider to be your vaccine efficacy, it is also important to know the risk of illness in the unvaccinated. Whether the risk in unvaccinated individuals is 0.8% or 0.00008%, the vaccine efficacy for the example above will still be 95%. So if a patient's risk of getting an infection or severe illness is 0.000001% but their risk of having an adverse reaction (that may include death or disability) is one hundred times higher than this (0.0001%), you should not be recommending the vaccine to them. Regardless of the RRR-based vaccine efficacy, if your individual risk must be considered before you get vaccinated. This is particularly important with the new mRNA vaccines and their unknown or questionable safety profiles. The mRNA vaccines should also never be compared to effective vaccines like the polio or smallpox vaccines. It's not only unprofessional to do so it's also a stark display of ignorance. Mandating the new mRNA vaccines in young children and women of reproductive age is questionable.

The recommendation to vaccinate young children under age 15 is not an evidence-based approach to care as pro-mRNA vaccine suitors tout and is likely not compassionate or ethical. Why? According to the *American Association of Pediatrics* data posted on services.aap.org as of June 10, 2021, there have been a total of 4,008,572 Covid-19 cases in children. This number represents 14.1% of all the 28 million plus cases. Severe Covid-19 illness is rare in children, and hospitalization and death an uncommon event. According to the same report, only 0.1-1.9% of all child Covid-19 cases resulted in hospitalization. Childhood Covid-19 deaths by state were 0.00% - 0.23%. Eight states in the USA reported no Covid-19 deaths in children. In the 43 states including New York City, Guam, and Puerto Rico, reporting on Covid-19 deaths in children, Covid-19 cases resulted in 0.00%-0.03% of deaths.

In the Forbes.com October article *What is Your Risk of Dying From Covid-19?* Getting infected with Covid-19 multiplies a 70-year old person's risk of death by 140%. That risk goes up by only six percent in people less than 20 years old. In Avik Roy's January 27, 2021 article on the freeopp.org website, the numbers are even more pronounced. According to Avik, a Covid-19 patient who is eighty-five years or older is 119 times more likely to die than a 25 to 34 year old while the same 25-34 year old is 73 times more likely to die than a child less than 15 years old. This simply means that a 14-year old child is 8,687 times less likely to die following Covid-19 infection, compared to an 85-year old, and 73 times less likely to die than a 25-34 year old. There is still no medical justification for vaccinating these young children. Except there is a hidden agenda or it's just plain corporate greed with total disregard for true efficacy. Again, I must emphasize that I am not anti-vaccine. The risk of harm outweighs the benefits of mRNA vaccines to children and mRNA vaccines should never be compared to effective immunization benefits from tetanus, measles, smallpox or polio. We must apply the brakes on vaccinating children with these new vaccines. If we don't then the policy makers may be psychopaths for allowing this to take place.

95% Vaccine Efficacy? Who Said That!

You're about to see another real life example of why this redundant or outright deceptive practice of using RRR-based vaccine efficacy calculations needs to be stopped globally. In at least two of the published clinical trials for the new Pfizer/BNT and Moderna mRNA vaccines, the difference between vaccinated and unvaccinated subjects was less than 1.2%. You probably have heard that these vaccines have an efficacy of 94 to 95 percent. This may be a bold misrepresentation that while legal may still be unethical. For example, in the Pfizer/BNT clinical trial, 99.25% of the unvaccinated placebo patients did not get infected with Covid-19. Let's use a simple illustration. Suppose you were hired to analyze the results of the Pfizer clinical trial and to find out how many subjects did not get infected in the placebo group. You were told the placebo group was vaccine B. You were so excited once you realized that vaccine B was really very effective and couldn't wait to submit your report the very next day. Vaccine B protected 99.25% of the recipients from Covid-19 you informed your supervisor. You notice your supervisor was however not as excited as you were. You went during your lunch break to find out why. She simply told you she wasn't excited because Vaccine B was a placebo! A very low infection rate of 0.75% left 99.25% uninfected. Such a high number in the untreated group leaves very little squeeze room for the Pfizer/BNT vaccine to claim a significant difference. Even if the mRNA vaccine were 100 percent effective, the difference between such a vaccine and the 99.25% in the placebo group (Vaccine B) in preventing infection would be a meager 0.75%. RRR is a way to get around this extremely small difference between placebo and vaccine.

Proper representation of the results of treatments in clinical trials can be done using relative risk reduction (RRR) odds ratio (OR), absolute risk reduction (ARR), or number needed to treat (NNT). Experts have chosen the last one, number needed to treat (NNT), as the best tool for evaluating treatments in clinical trials. (*Laupacis., et al, N. Engl. J. Med. 318: 1728, 1988*). That's what should be used in determining whether or not the new mRNA vaccines are helpful and to what extent. Arguing against this is pointless and at the same time revealing.

Number Needed To Treat: Pfizer/BNT and Moderna

The number needed to treat (NNT) is the reciprocal of the absolute risk reduction (1/ARR). In turn, the absolute risk reduction is the absolute difference between the treated (vaccinated) and untreated (placebo) groups.

For the Pfizer/BNT vaccine clinical trials reported in the December 10, 2020 issue of the New England Journal of Medicine, the absolute difference in the incidence of Covid-19 infection between the vaccinated group and unvaccinated groups can easily be calculated.

Of the 21,720 Pfizer mRNA vaccine recipients, 8 developed Covid-19.
Incidence of Covid-19 infections in vaccinated group =
Number of infected subjects/Number receiving vaccine
= (8/21720) x 100%
= **0.037%** (*Infected after Pfizer/BNT vaccine*)

Of the 21,728 placebo recipients in the Pfizer study, 162 developed Covid-19.
Incidence of Covid-19 infections in placebo group subjects =
Number of infected subjects/Number receiving placebo
= (162/21728) x 100%
= **0.75%** (*Infected after Pfizer placebo*)

The absolute difference in the incidence of Covid-19 infection between the vaccinated and unvaccinated placebo groups in the Pfizer study is therefore the difference between these two numbers:
0.75% - 0.037% = 0.713%

For the Pfizer vaccine trials therefore, the absolute risk reduction (ARR) between the vaccinated and unvaccinated groups, expressed as a number not a percentage, is **0.713% divided by 100%, or 0.00713.**

ARR for Pfizer/BNT vaccine trial = 0.00713.
1/ARR for Pfizer/BNT vaccine trial = 1/0.00713
1/ARR Pfizer =140
NNT for Pfizer vaccine = 140

Let's do the same calculations for the Moderna Vaccine trials:

Of the 15,210 Moderna mRNA vaccine recipients, 11 developed Covid-19.
Incidence of Covid-19 infections in vaccinated group
= Number of infected subjects/Number receiving vaccine
= (11/15,210) x 100%
= **0.072%** (*Infected after Moderna vaccine*)

Of the 15,210 placebo recipients in the Moderna study, 185 developed Covid-19.
Incidence of Covid-19 infections in placebo group subjects
= Number of infected subjects/Number receiving placebo
= (185/15,210) x 100%
= **1.22%** (*Infected after Moderna placebo*)

The absolute difference in the incidence of Covid-19 infection between the vaccinated and unvaccinated groups in the Moderna study is therefore the difference between these two numbers:
1.22% - 0.075% = 1.145%

For the Moderna vaccine trials therefore, the absolute risk reduction (ARR) between the vaccinated and unvaccinated groups, expressed as a number not a percentage, is **1.145% divided by 100% or 0.0114**

ARR for Moderna vaccine trial = 0.0114
1/ARR for Moderna vaccine trial = 1/0.0114 = 87.7
1/ARR Moderna= 88
NNT for Moderna mRNA vaccine =88

The absolute risk reduction number is not in a readily usable form for the average practicing healthcare professional. (Sackett et al, 1991). If you're trying to evaluate the benefit of a treatment and make a treatment decision based on a clinical trial, you need something more practical. The recommendations of experts in clinical epidemiology for evaluating the benefit of a treatment in a clinical trial is to use the number needed to treat (NNT), that is the reciprocal of the ARR. Why is this? According to Sackett et al, The NNT has several advantages:

> 1. The NNT is based on the absolute differences between the treatment groups, and accurately informs the practitioner on the clinical significance of the trial results and not just statistical significance.

> 2. The NNT tells us the number of patients we need to treat to prevent one complication of the disease. This is an important factor for evaluating the usefulness of the treatment.

> 3. The NNT also gives us a baseline for determining the costs of treatment as well as the cost of the side effects of treatment, if there are any.

> 4. The NNT helps in determining the clinical significance of a clinical trial where an event either happens or does not happen. In this instance, does the subject get Covid-19 infection or not?

> 5. The NNT helps the practitioner decide who to treat and who not to.

> 6. The NNT is therefore an extremely meaningful tool that can be rapidly used in making treatment decisions based on published clinical trial articles. It saves time and serves as a laser knife cutting through the maze of statistical data that may distort the one thing clinicians need to know, whether or not to treat or hold off on treatment based on the trial results.

A chart showing different baseline risks and their corresponding relative risk reductions can be helpful in determining NNT and the book *Clinical Epidemiology* has two such charts. NNT can also be calculated from the ARR if the latter number is available from clinical trials.

The ARR for the Pfizer/BNT mRNA vaccine clinical trials as calculated above is 0.00713. The NNT for the Pfizer/BNT vaccine trial is therefore 140. What is the significance of this? The NNT is the number of patients you will need to treat to get the desired effect in one patient. The ideal NNT is 1. That means if you treat one patient with the drug you will see a treatment effect in that single patient. If the NNT is 4 for example, it means that for you to get the desired treatment effect in one patient, you will have to treat 4 patients. A higher NNT means you have to treat more patients to get a benefit in a single patient. According to a March 2006 article (Chong et al, *Journal of Clinical Epidemiology,* 2006), NNT is a moderately accurate predictor of treatments that provide large health benefits. The article also showed that an NNT of 5 or lower is considered a favorable number for treating patients while an NNT greater than 15 had a sensitivity of 82% to 100% in ruling out therapies with low quality of life year. In other words, if the NNT is greater than 20, you're not getting the benefits easily. What about an NNT of 50, 80, 100, or an NNT of 140 like the Pfizer vaccine? If the risk of severe adverse events including death is high, or if these adverse events are under-reported or suppressed reports by the media, such a vaccine should not be forced on those who do not want it. Science is not tyranny and if statistics does not support such a vaccine, it should not be given outside of clinical trials. Some might argue that absolute risk reduction is not applicable to the pandemic or to vaccines. The same could however be said of relative risk reduction as it overinflates what vaccines can or cannot do.

Yet, we know how effective measles, smallpox and polio vaccines have been in eradicating the respective infections globally. Do the mRNA vaccines have the same efficacy? I don't think the mRNA vaccines should be compared to these other vaccines. Anyone with doubts about the safety of these newer mRNA vaccines is sane and a cognitively intact critical thinker. To be skeptic about getting the vaccine shows a level of sanity in an insane world. Are there improved patient outcomes following vaccination that cannot be explained by biases in assembly of study patients, or interpretation of responses to vaccination? If all the clinically relevant outcomes are measured, would the vaccine group fair better than the placebo group? For example, with the increasing number of serious adverse effects, development of myocarditis in younger children, and even death, do the risks not outweigh the benefits in children? In the Pfizer study, the vaccinated group does have a 12.5% mortality amongst those infected with Covid-19 while only 5.5% of those infected with Covid-19 in the placebo group died. Is that a clinically relevant piece of data? Was it overlooked? Is that why more are dying after receiving the vaccine?

While the vaccines may have some efficacy, it would be blatant misuse of statistics to claim 94 to 95 % efficacy for vaccines with a NNT greater than 10. In this case, the NNT's for both vaccines show a lack of efficacy. Hopefully, investigators will get to the bottom of this insistent misuse of statistics.

Statistics must be used in an ethical manner when interpreting and publishing data on the effectiveness of any treatments. Misrepresentation should be considered illegal. From what we have experienced during this pandemic, it is clear that data can be manipulated to a point where dangerously misleading material published in reputable journals, affects nations and billions of people. There should be international law governing the reporting and interpretation of clinical trials with punitive consequences for violators. Even more importantly, medical students and residents should receive more instruction time to learn how statistics can be used (medical students) or abused (residents) respectively. To understand how far Big Pharma can go, look up Professor Leemon McHenry's interview,

"Perspectives on The Pandemic. The Illusion of Evidence Based Medicine. Episode 13."

Chapter Z!

FDA's Fast Track Vaccine Authorization

The current mRNA vaccines came on the market without undergoing all the rigorous steps normally required for drug approvals by the FDA. Instead, a shortcut or fast track was followed due to the pandemic to bring the vaccine quickly to the market place. This requires that the FDA grant vaccine manufacturers a temporary go ahead called the Emergency Use Authorization (EUA). The EUA is granted to promising vaccines or drugs for use in certain emergency conditions. Drugs brought to consumers via the EUA are either brand new or old. The older drugs could either have been approved for specific conditions or may be in clinical trials for some time without FDA approval for any specific conditions. These older drugs, whether approved or not, usually have an established safety profile. If an urgent indication is found for the unapproved drug, it is easy to bring it to the market place through an EUA, since it's safety is already known. To get the EUA, a vaccine or drug must still meet the following FDA criteria:

1. A Serious or Life-Threatening Condition
2. Evidence of Effectiveness
3. Benefit Outweighs Risks of the Disease or Treatment
4*. No Alternative

Vaccine manufacturers for SARS-CoV-2 can meet the first three conditions easily. For the first condition, we have a killer pandemic. For the second, data has been created using statistics to show effectiveness. Based on clinical trials, vaccine manufacturers have also presented safety and efficacy data that appear to meet the third condition. The fourth condition however requires that there be **no other alternative treatments.** If there is an available alternative treatment such as hydroxychloroquine or ivermectin, the mRNA vaccines cannot get the EUA from the FDA. That's why early treatments don't work in US Covid-19 patients! These treatments do work in Covid-19 patients outside the USA! Not funny. These other countries do not have an FDA regulation demanding a fourth condition. So they gladly welcome early treatments as well as mRNA vaccines. I'm sure we wouldn't have had this many deaths and so much animosity between doctors if this fourth condition did not exist. Perhaps there would not have been this many deaths if the CDC and NIH had accurately instructed doctors on exactly how to use hydroxychloroquine and ivermectin. The fourth criteria for obtaining an EUA should be modified to accommodate vaccine manufacturers in the future. That way, patients can get already available, inexpensive, alternative treatments with established safety profiles while manufacturers continue working on creating needed even though expensive vaccines.

This "No Alternative" 4th criterion in the forty-nine page document by the FDA and U.S Department of Health and Human Services titled *Emergency Use Authorization of Medical Products and Related Authorities: Guidance for Industry and Other Stakeholders* and dated January 2017 states on page 8 that

"For FDA to issue an EUA, there must be no adequate, approved, and available alternative to the candidate product for diagnosing, preventing, or treating the disease condition".

This fourth condition obviously stood in the way of the current mRNA vaccine manufacturers. Removing this fourth condition would have been a win-win situation for everyone. Or would it? Unless the fourth condition was added by the influential mRNA vaccine manufacturers themselves! Perhaps they thought they would be first to reach the finish line for creating a covid-19 magic bullet. The 4th condition would have conveniently blocked all their competitors after they came up with the Covid-19 magic bullet. Unfortunately, that same 4th condition that was meant to block their competitors was now blocking them.

There are major players that make up the *Covid-19 Industrial Complex*. They might be responsible for the development and spreading of the SARS-CoV-2 virus and creating this pandemic. They have the money and political clout and can operate at any policy-shaping level of government. That will be the only theory that explains the arrant behaviors of the officials at the NIH, CDC, FDA and WHO. It may also explain the behaviors of medical journalism terrorists as well as the current battle amongst scientists and healthcare professionals over treatments and methodology at the expense of people's lives.

We might have a money and power greedy group co-sponsoring the development of a deadly virus on the one hand, and hoping to bring a magic cure to the market on the other hand. They will make trillions of dollars, while putting in place an FDA guidance clause #4, that hinders the competition from joining the feast. Alas, HCQ beat them to the treatment line and it had to be murdered or martyred. It reads like a Hollywood movie script, doesn't it? This may be the undisclosed truth behind the entire pandemic and the Covid-19 industrial complex stemming from it. While still unlikely, and I'm hoping the human race has not sunk this low, it still cannot be entirely ruled out. If this is true, then the special interests group(s) desiring the spread of SARS-CoV-2 in order to profit through vaccines and treatments will not want the pandemic to end. Disallowing any early "unproven" treatments was the only way to sustain the pandemic and the EUA. Otherwise these "unproven" treatments could wipe out the entire pandemic, leaving nothing left for the Covid-

19 "magic bullet" to eliminate and no heroes in the sponsor camps. If this is true, then this group may have invested millions or even billions to pull off this seemingly sinister plan. So even when the vaccine efficacy and safety is questioned, they keep moving their plans forward. How? By buying the political influence of a few powerful government officials. What if their plan is to hit the rich economy of the USA with both viruses and vaccines and make four to twelve trillion dollars? And what if they intend to release deadly variants of these viruses intermittently, requesting more mandatory vaccinations every three to nine months, and sell these new vaccines? If this is the plan, then the human race is in far more trouble than the current pandemic suggests. Even if there are alternatives to treating Covid-19, a group of decision makers in government are pretending they don't exist. They act as if these alternatives are more dangerous than the vaccine or the virus. They simply ignore the available data and the doctors requesting the use of early treatment alternatives. From all that we've seen so far, this looks like an ironclad plan that has been put to work. If the goal is to sell trillions of dollars of vaccines to the rich governments around the world, who is going to stop them? Making money, lots of it is not a crime. Doing so at the expense of human lives while using unsafe treatments with high incidences of severe adverse events and pretending to be benevolent at the same time is a serious legal and ethical problem. That's why you must understand these remedies.

In September 2020, I estimated 4.3 trillion dollars for a **Covid-19** *magic bullet* in my book *The HCQ Debate: What Did Researchers Hide.* That meant they had to find a ways to prevent any alternative treatments from reaching those affected, in order to get the EUA for their new vaccines. It shouldn't surprise you why some US government officials are fighting vehemently to ignore or avoid recommending any early safe, inexpensive treatments for Covid-19 till today. They consistently issued policy statements that totally ignored these potentially useful treatments. Acknowledging such early treatments, would wipe out any chances of any Covid-19 vaccine receiving emergency use authorization. Trillions of dollars in potential profits for Big Pharma would be lost. We know the drugs used for the treatment of early Covid-19 work outside the USA and are safe. They already have FDA approval for other conditions and have an established and impressive safety profile spanning decades of use with billions of prescriptions.

Safety for the mRNA vaccines does not come close to that of the proposed alternative early treatments. As a matter of fact, there have been enough problems with the vaccines recently that demand a vaccine recall. According to the CDC.gov website, the swine flu led to 1 case of Guillaine-Barre Syndrome (GBS) for every 100,000 people that got the Swine flu vaccine in 1976. Guillain-Barre Syndrome is a serious neurological disorder that that simulates severe spinal cord injury. It can lead to muscle paralysis and death. After over 40 million people were vaccinated with this vaccine, federal health officials decided that no matter how small the association of this vaccine with GBS was, it was time to stop. They stopped.

How do vaccine manufacturers get away with the attacks on early treatments, particularly when lives are at stake? Except for Merck attacking its own ivermectin, Big Pharma simply pays stooges to do their dirty work. Doctors, instructors, journalists, college professors, politicians, community leaders and politicians all working together help spread the "right" message.

You'd be naïve and wrong to think government officials are only concerned with scientific data and are not influenced by private entities like vaccine manufacturers. Between 1999 and 2018, Big Pharma paid about $233 million dollars every year to senators and lawmakers, according to Dr. Olivier Wouters' March 3, 2020 article in the Journal of the American Medical Association *JAMA Internal Medicine*. That came to $4.7 billion dollars over twenty years. What does Big Pharma get in return?

In 2019 alone, the US Government spent $369.7 billion dollars on prescription drugs. That's a good return on Big Pharma's annual investment. The amount of money they hope to make from this pandemic is beyond human comprehension. I explained the breakdown cost of a *Covid-19 magic bullet* in *The HCQ Debate*. Nevertheless, just imagine you have an Uncle who makes one million dollars per hour from his multiple businesses. In one year, with 8760 hours in a year, your Uncle would have made $8.76 billion. It would take another 500 years for him to make $4.38 trillion dollars. What if instead of making one million dollars an hour, we multiply what your uncle makes in one hour by 500 so that he can make what he would have made in 500 years in one year? All your uncle has to do is make *$500 million dollars an hour* to get to $4.38 trillion dollars in one year. I recommend you read *The HCQ Debate* to get a grasp of why this pandemic is still with us today. It's the money!

Except some whistleblower reveals the deep secrets behind the *Covid-19 Industrial Complex* as someone wisely put it, Big Pharma intends to make trillions no matter how many die. That's one of the reasons you will continue to see outright attacks on these early treatments for now. If folk can kill for millions or billions, certainly for trillions, most will sell their soul to the devil! Unfortunately even academic physicians have joined this attacking bandwagon. In addition to the attacks on useful alternative treatments and the doctors recommending them by the mainstream media journalists, scientists have been fighting doctors treating Covid-19 patients with previously approved agents. We should not forget that the majority of scientists depend on grants and favors from the major players in the vaccine industry. Most don't make money from seeing patients or working directly with patients in clinics, emergency rooms or hospitals. Bureaucrats have also been busy creating bottlenecks to hinder doctors in the US and other developed countries like Australia and Canada. Add this to the silence of the US top infectious disease expert Dr. Fauci's silence about any early treatments besides expensive drugs and the failed Remdesivir (*I wrote about this inevitable failure and Trojan Horse in May 2020*), and you may see why we still have a pandemic. To top it all, several medical journalists have been feeding us with misinformation and intellectual graffiti over the last 17 months.

But you survived it all. Unfortunately surviving Covid-19 doesn't mean freedom from the aftermath of the infection. You may become a chronic Covid-19 long hauler. And no one except a few exceptional doctors will be willing to help you. It's clear there is still a great need for both remedies and treatments and not just vaccines. Yet the government is still silent about them. This is what happens when everyone that went to medical school gets to be called doctor, even when they have no iota of compassion for the human race. What's more important is that you must know how to take better care of yourself. If doctors, scientists and government officials can't agree on what's in your best interests, you should at least have information on what you can do for yourself and your loved ones. The healthcare system may not respond adequately to what you need in order to remain healthy or to heal. I wrote this book just for people like you who want to know what to do personally and collectively.

I have seen firsthand the negative impact of doctors arguing about methodology on the patients they swore to protect while the patients gradually slip way from the land of the living. Many of them end up hospitalized and eventually die. It's so much easier to read research papers and calculate p values and then argue with doctors facing real patients in real life who must decide what is best for their patients. I commend the doctors engaged in actively treating patients using evidence-based medicine in spite of the naysayers. We do know that randomized placebo controlled double blinded clinical trials (RCT) are the gold standard for treatment decisions. RCTs are however not the only component of evidence-based medicine. RCTs can also be manipulated at multiple points to make an effective drug seem useless (Ivermectin, HCQ,) and a useless one seem useful. (Remdesivir).

Randomized control tricks are randomized placebo-controlled double-blinded gold standard clinical trials intentionally designed to ensure the outcomes are exactly what the pharmaceutical companies want. Many of the agents for early treatment of Covid-19 failed not because the drugs were ineffective. They failed because they were designed by special interest groups to fail. (*The HCQ Debate*). That way, vaccines can remain the only option. The mRNA vaccines designed to prevent infection, unlike effective tetanus immunizations, have now been shown to not prevent infection. That's why you still had to wear a mask after getting vaccinated. As a result of this primary failure of the mRNA vaccines in preventing infection, the pharmaceutical companies adopted the **Texas Sharp Shooter fallacy**. This fallacy refers to shooting first, then drawing circles around the bullet holes in order to look like an expert shot. What the vaccine manufacturers set out to do has become a moving target. When you look at hard end points like reduction in hospitalization, transmission, length of hospitalization, deaths, intubations, the vaccine does no better than what early treatment trials using much cheaper "alternatives" have shown. So whatever they say the vaccine does is after the fact, a moving target. The efficacy data for early treatments with HCQ and several other drugs accompanied by a better safety profile have been impressive. Yet the desire of Big Pharma is to spread negative results in order force vaccines on everyone. The NNTs for these vaccines is quite high, the adverse effects are unacceptable.

I AM NOT ANTIVAX but will not support what looks like an Orwellian instrument of oppression. The vaccine has untoward side effects and violates what I signed up for as a doctor to support. More so, there are safer alternatives. The vaccine manufacturers could not answer simple questions of efficacy and duration, and whether or not natural antibodies can protect following infection with the virus itself. They don't even want antibodies measured in those that may have been previously exposed. We know there is a real danger of antibody-derived enhancement (ADE) of infection. Could this phenomenon explain the unusually high incidence of deaths and serious adverse effects like myocarditis in young vaccine recipients? Drug manufacturers are not trying to figure out why these patients are dying within a short period after vaccination. Instead, they're trying to cover their tracks. When healthy twenty, thirty or forty year olds die within days of getting the mRNA vaccine, what do manufacturers do? They have a spokesperson come out and tell the media they have looked into it and do not believe the vaccine caused the death of these healthy victims. When an adverse event including death is connected to the temporal sequence of exposure to a specific agent, what should be done? Halt the use of the agent! Instead they're trying to make the same agent a mandatory administration to enter businesses buses or burger shops. This is insanity. of a correlates with the death Everything we've done for patients so far has been based on sound moral code and ethics, dedication to caring for the human body soul and spirit, as well as taking the Hippocratic oath. Doctors want to do far more to help their patients than they are usually able to do. Unlike doctors, the drug companies don't have a Hippocratic oath to adhere to. They just make money regardless of whatever pain and suffering they cause families, individuals or even communities. Again, I recommend you watch the YouTube video *"The Illusion of Evidence Based Medicine"* interview with Professor Leemon McHenry. You'll see how Big Pharma has corrupted the most reputable medical journals. These are the same journals we are expected to trust for decisions on new drugs. The trust I have for these journals before the pandemic has turned into skepticism. That trust we doctors have has been abused thoroughly that there is hardly anything left to trust about pharmaceutical companies. For example, while Vioxx Rofecoxib was causing increased incidence of strokes and heart attacks, the FDA and the drug manufacturers ignored the warnings. A group of cardiologists even came out with a paper denouncing the assertions that Rofecoxib increased stroke and heart attack risk. How could they do that, or more specifically did they really write the paper themselves? It is quite common today for pharmaceutical companies to hire a medical writer to create a research paper to counter true research or to say exactly what the pharmaceutical company wants them to. Everything can be geared towards marketing a specific drug or device or attack a rival drug. Results are tailored to meet the desires of the drug company. The writer hands the paper back to the pharmaceutical company representative who then finds the appropriate doctors to pay and have their name glued on the paper. I was surprised to learn about this fraudulent behavior from Professor Leemon McHenry. Doctors are paid to put their good name on a paper created by someone else and the paper is finalized by the drug company and published in top notch medical journals! Influential professors, academicians and doctors, are usually sought. If caught, the paper is retracted, but that doesn't happen very often. You should therefore be more discerning when reading medical journals if you're a healthcare professional. This is very important when looking at new treatments. I guess that's one more reason our attending physicians during residency insisted we learn how to critically evaluate the medical literature. Wolf in sheep clothing have infiltrated our profession and are using trusted platforms and our reliance on them to destroy the honesty and integrity in the medical profession. That's probably why today, our compassionate caring profession of patient care has been turned into the business of health care where profits are more important than patients, the cash register more than caring. Have you noticed that healthcare in America is first about business care, money care, and not patient care? The journals and our medical societies will have to work really hard to regain the trust of critically thinking doctors.

Beneficence is treating people in an ethical manner, respecting their decisions and protecting them from harm. If the vaccine is more likely to harm you than to help you, giving you the vaccine is not beneficence. A doctor prescribing it to you if the risk outweighs its benefit is doing something wrong. Getting such a new vaccine without receiving written **informed consent** is in violation of the ethical principles of *The Belmont Report*, a document prepared by the Department of Health and Human Services. (hhs.gov). Going to a drive-through and getting jabbed with the Covid-19 vaccine by an unknown person without a doctor signing an informed consent with you might actually be illegal. It also means you can't prove you were injured by the vaccine even if you have proof you received the vaccine.

In addition, vaccine manufacturers have ironclad immunity against vaccine injuries. The way they are brushing off vaccine injuries with an obvious temporal sequence following its administration in victims, they seem to have zero liability for the mRNA vaccines. Doctors recommending the vaccine on the other hand are at risk of being sued for recommending the vaccine to patients or the general public. Somebody has to be sued and I would hate for my colleagues to become victims of a monster they did not create. If an employer insists that a critical employee get the vaccine and that employee develops and dies or becomes disabled from an adverse reaction, who is held responsible. According to the *Council for International Organizations of Medical Sciences* (CIOMS) 2017 *Guide to Active Vaccine Safety Surveillance,* passive reporting of adverse events following immunization (AEFI) is the responsibility of the healthcare provider. AEFI's are underreported, and in the absence of active physician involvement may not be reliable. Active Vaccine Safety Surveillance (AVSS) is now necessary with the significant reports obtained of AEFIs. There is a significant knowledge gap (SKG) regarding the risk vs. benefit for a significant population and that risk is been ignored: the young, and those with previous SARS-CoV-2 infection and may be at risk of developing ADE of infection. To date , there re no numbers r any sound research on the risk of ADE following vaccination. The goal is to just blindly vaccinate everyone. That's not science. They hope to answer these questions presented to them only after they have obtained sufficient data from the population vaccinated. That in effect makes administering these vaccines experimentation, even if it is not research. It's beginning to fit into the Nuremberg pattern of events. Germans trusted their government and that led to the concentration camps. This administering of mRNA vaccines with severe adverse effects of this nature particularly in young children is no longer science or beneficence. It is now looking more like a Gestapo tactic fueled by greed. How far will it go before it is stopped? beyond what has currently been carried out appears to violate The Belmont Report provides guidelines for protecting human subjects of research. The recipients of this new vaccine are in experimentation but unless the vaccine manufacturers admit they are researching their vaccine recipients through this mass vaccination, it doesn't qualify as research. The ethical principles are unchanged regardless of whether this act is research or experimentation. The continued administration of these vaccines particularly to young children, even when the risk outweigh the benefits is indicative of a need to remedy the current laws and regulations. It's almost certain that we will soon start finding research papers from prominent academicians showing that there s no link between mRNA vaccines and myocarditis in young vaccine recipients. Such a paper will probably come from "recent studies" from leading researchers from three different parts of the world or three different institutions, all about the same time. The Vaccine Safety Net (VSN), Vaccine Adverse Event Reporting System, (VAERS), WHO, and FDA, CDC, NIH, most pharmaceutical companies and the different medical journals and News channels on television networks were all set up for good intentions. Can you vouch for all of them today? How many have been tainted? Injecting people with high-risk mRNA vaccines may not fall under the full jurisdiction of the Belmont Report since jabbing people without informed consent at some pharmacy or drive through is no longer research but experimentation. But perhaps, there is still a remedy for the impending insanity.

Vaccines are generally safe. Nevertheless, skepticism against the new mRNA vaccines should never be considered an anti-vaccine position. It's a healthy skepticism by any clearly thinking person. A lack of any skepticism against these new vaccines without any track record of safety is actually detrimental to balance in a civilized society. It means we have all accepted Big Pharma's propaganda that drugs can solve every human problem. That would be a poor reflection of our ability to think critically as human beings. Thank God that's not the case. Those against vaccines in general may have an anti-vaccine axe to grind. That anti-vaccine position does not necessarily apply to those who think the new vaccines are unsafe. There are logical reasons to think so. And then there are early treatments that work.

What's happening now is Orwellian. Science has been bought and paid for by Big Pharma. While the massive budget of the NIH to support scientific research from tax dollars gave out $31 billion in research funding in 2011, Big Pharma spent a whopping $39 billion, according to Peter Whoriskey's *November 24, 2012 Washington Post* article. Most academic and medical research centers around the world benefit from these two sources of funding and will do whatever they're told to do. That's why we keep getting conflicting information from our trusted, academic, healthcare, and government institutions and individuals on Covid-19. These institutions and trusted individuals tainted by Big Pharma have no intentions of publishing the truth about HCQ, Ivermectin or other alternatives, any time soon.

In the latter part of this second edition, I have shared my strange experience, a series of events that happened less than 48 hours after I announced that the first edition of this book was available to the public. Amazon refused to publish it and blocked it. The ensuing drama and few other strange events afterwards are described in chapters 22 and 23. I personally don't like drama so I have kept it all towards the end. If you love drama, you can go straight to it. The last chapter is dedicated to inspiring you to your own greatness.

REMEDY 1

HOT PEPPERS!

Whenever the flu season arrives and once exposed to the flu, some of my good friends have judiciously increased their intake of hot peppers in their food. Some use ground cayenne pepper, others would just get hot jalapeno peppers or grind it up in their foods. I have seen it recommended for those down with a really bad cold only to find them at work the next day and thanking the powers of hot "Nigerian" pepper soup. But would such peppers work with this ongoing pandemic? Or is it insane to expect that in the face of nothing else available, we should try cayenne or jalapeno peppers or something similar or even hotter? If we don't, are we doing everything we can that could work? The US Surgeon General, Vice Admiral Adams, said on television early after the pandemic was declared

"We cannot hold back on trying everything that could work, particularly if it's safe to do so."

That's the spirit! In the face of this horrible pandemic that's how to go. I have fallen victim to really bad colds when worn out by my hectic emergency room and hospital medicine schedules. I found to my surprise, that hot peppers do really have strange, safe, but consistent healing powers. In the case of the flu, once the symptoms have been going on for more than 4 days, it is too late to give Tamiflu. So what should you do if you've had flu symptoms for more than 4 days and are no longer a candidate for Tamiflu? You can take hot pepper soup if you can handle the hot spicy pepper. I have seen and experienced phenomenal results with hot peppers in my food whenever I come down with the flu once the symptoms start. What's more important is that there is an ingredient responsible for the antiviral effect of hot peppers, and it's called capsaicin. Capsaicin is the active ingredient responsible for the hotness of hot peppers and has been shown to have antiviral, antioxidant, anti-inflammatory and analgesic effects. Capsaicin is a possible option for those exposed to any viral infection. The following scientific evidence might help you understand this chemical better.

In the November 2015 issue of *Frontiers in Microbiology* by Emanuela Marini and colleagues from Italy, capsaicin was shown to have both anti-virulence and antimicrobial activity against a highly invasive strain of Group A Streptococci that was already resistant to erythromycin. Capsaicin prevented the bacteria from invading the cells. There must be a biochemical process not yet fully studied responsible for the neutralizing effect of capsaicin on bacteria and viruses. In the October 1992 issue of the journal of *Medical Virology*, Dr. Lawrence Stanberry and colleagues also reported that capsaicin helped reduce the severity of herpes simplex virus infection by preventing the spread of the herpes virus.

If you're infected or exposed to viral infections, increasing your intake of peppers may be very helpful and in instances where there is no detectable causal agent, one of your few real options for healing. You can add dried ground pepper to your food or soups, or make a broth with hot peppers. Be sure your digestive tract can handle the pepper lest you end up at the doctor's for a heartburn or anal burning diarrhea!

For fear of being seen as quacks, many a doctor may sneer at you for using hot peppers even when they don't have anything else to offer you. So recognize that there is a scientific basis for how peppers work. Use it when you have to. Just make sure you can handle it.

REMEDY 2

TABLE SALT

Highly concentrated table salt solution can be used to gargle in order to kill the microorganisms in the mouth and the throat. The cells exposed to the high concentrations of salt in the throat as you gargle will lose water by osmosis and become dehydrated. The scientific term is called crenation. As the cells lose water, they shrink. As they shrink, their protective cell wall can become distorted enough to allow the super-concentrated salt solution to leak into the organism. The genetic material in these organisms, whether DNA or RNA, is sensitive to dehydration and can become damaged from dehydration and exposure to the highly concentrated salt solution leaking into the cells from your throat. Death or inactivation follows and sometimes that's all you'll need to do in order to fight an early invasion by bacteria or viruses. Your immune system will take care of the rest. Of course a late invasion with bacteria multiplying heavily will lead to pharyngitis and perhaps even a fever that may require a throat swab and antibiotics. So whenever you start having symptoms such as a sore throat, particularly following suspected exposure, you should immediately place a teaspoonful of table salt into 4 tablespoons of warm water and gargle with it. Then consult your doctor right away.

This is not recommended for little children at risk of choking or debilitated adults who might aspirate. Gargle with the concentrated salt solution for about 30 seconds and spit it out. Repeat this at least twice and wait for about 5 minutes after your third gargle before rinsing your mouth. This will allow the concentrated salt solution to attack the genetic material of the virus or bacteria in your throat. You can do this three times a day for the next two days. Don't swallow the salt. You should get relief and such relief has a scientific basis: intracellular killing of bacteria as well as reducing neutrophil induced inflammatory cytokine release and the accompanying tissue destruction. (*Shields et al., Annals of Surgery, Volume 238, Number 2, August 2003*). Chloride ions have also been shown to inhibit cell inflammatory destruction induced by interleukin IL-1β, probably by repressing P2X7R activation of caspase-1 induced IL-1β production. (*Verhoef PA, et al., J Immunol December 1, 2005, 175(11):7623-7634*). Mucus plugs can lead to lung collapse in Covid-19 patients, creating an emergency or life-threatening situation. Inhaled hypertonic saline (5ml of a 7% solution) increases mucus clearance in patients with cystic fibrosis and it might do the same for you. (*Donaldson HS et al., N Engl J Med. January 19, 2006 354:3:241-250*). The ELVIS (Edinburgh Lothians Viral Intervention Study) of 66 adults by the British National Health Service evaluated the effect of nasal saline irrigation on viral inhibition. Coronaviruses (CoV-B3, HCoV 229E) as well as herpes simplex virus, RSV, Influenza A were all inhibited in a dose dependent manner and a reduction in duration of symptoms of upper respiratory infection of 2 days. (*Ramalingam S., et al., Scientific Reports 8, 2018:1-11; Ramalingam S., et al., Scientific Reports 9, 1015 2019*). Since higher viral loads of SARS-CoV-2 were detected in nasal swabs compared with throat swabs, (*Zou l., et al., N Engl J Med 2020; 382:1177-9*) hypertonic saline nasal irrigation and nebulized saline using ultrasonic humidifiers (*Le, Nguyen, Wilkinson et al., Immunome Res, 2020; Vol.17 Iss.1 No:185*) can be a very effective remedy. There's no reason to think hypertonic saline would be any less effective in SARS-CoV-2. Shrinking and destruction of the cell wall or viral coat can also be a direct consequence of direct contact with hypertonic saline.

REMEDY 3

MENTHOLS

Vapor Rub, eucalyptus oil and menthols, applied topically to the skin and your mucosal surfaces may be helpful for painful, itchy hemorrhoids, colds, flu-like symptoms as well as body aches and pains. Some will apply menthol balms to the joints to relieve mild or moderate symptoms of arthritis, to the chest wall for acute bronchitis and the flu and they obtain relieve. The older parents of many physicians probably used these menthol rubs to relieve their aching joints and mild upper respiratory infections but very few if any of us took the time to understand how they work or if they were just placebos. I suppose we presumed the latter. Both my grandmothers used these chest balms, Robb®, Vicks®, Mentholatum® and the likes regularly. My paternal grandmother lived to be eighty-six and my maternal grandmother one hundred years. Walmart's Equate™ brand has a chest rub consisting of a combination of 4.8% camphor listed as a cough suppressant and topical analgesic, 1.2% eucalyptus oil, listed as a cough suppressant, and 2.6% menthol, listed as a cough suppressant and topical analgesic on its label. It is unclear to many how these chest rubs work, and I thought I would have a really hard time explaining how they work or to find convincing scientific proof, no matter how small. In the December 2003 issue of the *Journal of Ethnopharmacology*, Jeane Silva and colleagues reported analgesic effects to hot plate stimulation in rats after administering *Eucalyptus (E) citridora, E. teraticornis E. globulus* extracts. They also found a reduction in rat paw edema induced by carrageenan and dextran irritants. They basically burnt rat paws and gave them eucalyptus applications that relieved the pain. While inconsistencies where found that could be attributed to assay methods, the study showed that eucalyptus oil extracts do have a combination of analgesic and anti-inflammatory effects. This means that if you have mild symptoms or are exposed to Covid-19 infected individuals but have no symptoms, applying the chest rub might be beneficial. With the ongoing pandemic, hospitals expect reasonably healthy though Covid-19 positive patients to self-quarantine at home. Applying the chest rubs to your chest while at home, along with the many other remedies mentioned here in this book, may be far more helpful than just fearfully waiting at home, hopelessly wishing your Covid-19 infection won't get worse. It is far more likely that what you do after reading this book will be the only thing that can stop the progression of the infection to life threatening respiratory failure. Don't expect pharmaceutical companies to sponsor or publish any studies showing that a $3 chest rub will help you after you get infected with a potentially deadly illness like Covid-19. It's not going to happen.

In Chapter 21 of the book *Medicinal Plant Research in Africa* and titled *Anti-Oxidant Activity of African Medicinal Plants*, contributing authors Mikhail Nafiu, Musa Salawu, and Mutiu Kazeem, described *Eucalyptus calmadulensis* extracts as used for infections of the urinary and respiratory tract. The authors state that eucalyptus has anti-inflammatory, antibacterial properties as well as hydroxyl radical scavenging properties.

Eucalyptus oil poses a significant risk of toxicity particularly in children, as does camphor. So be sure to follow the manufacturer's guidelines on whatever you choose to use. Like all potential poisons, keep it away from children

Menthols and eucalyptus oils compounded to create such products as the Vicks Vapor Rub® do have a scientific basis for their folk remedy reputation. While physicians are apt to make a mockery of such remedies, including myself until the pandemic hit, the sole basis for such mockery itself may stem from pure ignorance. It's clear in today's world that available scientific data is often sponsored and made available by big pharmaceutical companies (aka Big Pharma) with loads of money. Therefore it is unlikely that any low-cost effective remedies would be presented to physicians as tenable options until randomized clinical trials are conducted. Guess who sponsors more than half of randomized control trials. It's Big Pharma! In this pandemic situation however, we don't have time and we need solutions immediately that will offload the overburdened healthcare system at all entry and exit points. England's Prime Minister Boris Johnson, my wife informed me just now, is in the intensive care unit. I pray that those caring for him can think outside the box.

REMEDY 4

STEAM INHALATION

Our body makes just over a liter of mucus daily beginning in the nose all the way down to the lungs. Mucus keeps the lining of the cells well-hydrated and protected from drying. It can also prevent bacteria, viruses and fungi from entering our bodies. When you inhale steam as in the steam baths often seen in old Mafia movies, you loosen the mucus. *The American Burn Association* has however issued directives to prevent you from burning yourself while performing steam inhalation. A much safer way to experience the benefits of water vapor on the airways is to sip hot soup. Not sure if this has a scientific basis? Hold tight. In the *Chest* journal of *October 1978 [74 (4), 408-410]*, Dr. K Saketkhoo and colleagues measured mucosal velocity and nasal airflow resistance in 15 healthy subjects, before as well as at 5 and 30 minutes after drinking hot water, hot chicken soup and cold water. In all three categories, subjects sipped the liquid directly from its container or sipped with a straw. Hot water sips increased nasal mucus velocity from 6.2mm per minute to 8mm/minute, hot chicken soup sips from 6.9 to 9.2mm/minute, and chicken soup by straw from 6.4 to 7.8mm per minute, five minutes after administration. All values returned to their baseline at 30 minutes except for cold water. Cold water decreased the mucosal velocity from the nasal mucus velocity from 7.3 to 4.5 mm per minute. There was no change in nasal airflow resistance at any time after the liquids were taken.

In a study reported in the 2001 issue of the *European Respiratory Journal*, Chivers and colleagues inoculated the nostrils of healthy volunteers with human corona virus HCoV 229E. By day 3 the ciliated epithelium was disrupted and the cilia would not move the way they should in these healthy volunteers. Three of the subjects did not have any symptoms. The researchers concluded that damage to the respiratory epithelium could occur without any real symptoms. This ciliary epithelial damage and movement malfunction induced by HCoV 229E means that clearing of mucus will be difficult in human corona virus (HCoV) infected patients. Perhaps that's why many Covid-19 patients don't have a troubling cough. The damaged lining of the airways may still produce mucus but it doesn't flow upward and outward to be coughed out due to the damaged ciliated epithelium. Warm humidified air can increase the slipperiness of the mucus and allow you to cough out the infected phlegm. But with corona virus damaging the lining of the lungs and air passages as mentioned above, you will need more effort to cough up the infected mucus or phlegm. Just make sure you do not ignore or downplay the symptoms that may start with a mild throat discomfort or itch that rapidly advances into a life-threatening pneumonia; you must act immediately.

You can also soak a clean hand towel in warm water and gently apply it over your nasal bridge and sinuses for some relief. Unfortunately, as soon as videos started appearing on the Internet, a particular US medical association, rather than tell people how to use steam inhalation safely, began posting warnings that steam inhalation can cause burns. Yet, the US Veterans Administrations has had a long-standing recommendation for veterans to inhale steam in order to open up their stuffy noses! Amazing.

REMEDY 5

COUGHING IT UP!

While gargling with warm salt water can kill the bugs in the back of your throat that are causing a pharyngitis, such an action can also loosen thick phlegm in the back of your throat. This thick phlegm stuck to the back of your throat may harbor live, actively multiplying bacteria, viruses, as well as cytokines. The cytokines can trigger local inflammation with pain and redness, as well as a more systemic fever and generalized body aches. You should therefore make some attempts to cough up the phlegm by first drinking enough warm water or soup. If you cough up mucus loaded with bacteria, viruses, or cytokines, you'll be getting rid of an otherwise rich source of millions of bacteria, viruses and cytokines that could make you sicker. You will also be clearing the airways to help you breath better. Inability to clear this mucus due to damaged ciliary epithelium may eventually lead to mucus plugging of the airways. This may present as cough, shortness of breath and wheezing. Guafenesin and other similar over the counter cough medicines may assist with clearing this cough as can the soothing effect of menthols found in many cough medicines.

In a study by Rodrigo Rodrigues *et al* published in the July 2002 issue of the journal of *Clinical and Diagnostic Laboratory Immunology*, patients with tuberculosis were found to have higher levels of interferon-gamma in their sputum compared to healthy subjects or those with bacterial pneumonia. If cytokine-laden mucus is present anywhere along the respiratory tract, it may still trigger fever, body aches, cough and shortness of breath. Therefore sputum needs to be coughed up and you should make every attempt to do so. Proper hydration by adequate intake of fluids will also help move the mucus forward and upward out of your airway passages.

The phlegm may be quite thick and should be coughed up quickly and regularly while staying well hydrated. Not coughing up the phlegm could result in plugging of the airways with hyaluronic acid-dense mucus plugs that can potentially completely cut off the airway. Hyaluronan absorbs about 1000 times its weight in water and the jelly-like material seen in Covid-19 lungs has been attributed to the high levels of hyaluronan. *(Yufang Shi et al, Cell Death and Differentiation 27, 1451-1454).*

Following suspected exposure to Covid-19, use the remedies, cough up and spit out as much phlegm, and as frequently as possible.

What you don't cough up may plug off your airways. The respiratory mucosal secretions have been shown to contain hyaluronic acid. This can become a sponge that absorbs a thousand times its weight in water. It can create an expanding foam sealant-like effect that suddenly cuts off air when it plugs the airway passages. So coughing up phlegm can become a life-saving maneuver.

REMEDY 6

GINGER

In the January 9, 2013 issue of the *Journal of Ethnopharmacology*, Dr. Chang and colleagues at Taiwan's University of Kaohsiung College of Medicine showed that fresh but not dried ginger (Zingiber officinale Roscoe), inhibited the attachment of respiratory syncytial virus, (RSV) to cells. RSV is a virus that commonly infects children under the age of two causing bronchiolitis and wheezing in the winter. It can lead to severe respiratory distress. As the 2015 article by Dr. RB Semwal in the September issue of the journal *Phytochemistry* suggests, the multiple chemical compounds found in ginger make it a potential candidate for developing multiple drugs due to their anti-oxidant, anti-cancer, antimicrobial, anti-allergic, and anti-inflammatory effects. In addition to these, ginger has been shown to possess free radical scavenging, nausea-reducing and gastric ulcer prevention properties in a June 2013 article by Haniadka et al published in *Food Function*. The immune-modulatory, lipid-lowering effects and anti-diabetic functions of ginger have equally been well-documented in journals such as Ali et al did in the February 2008 issue of *Food Chem Toxico.* Eat fresh ginger, especially if you think you might have been exposed to Covid-19.

REMEDY 7

LEMON PEEL

At first, I laughed when I saw the YouTube video of a Black lady with her head over a pot of steaming water and a cloth or towel over her head. Next to her was another adult female asking her how she felt after she had been on this "treatment" for about 5 minutes. She said she felt so much better. Sounded quite ridiculous until you decide to examine the objective facts. They weren't trying to sell anything and they didn't look like they owned a citrus farm either. The lady next to the one getting the steam therapy went on to describe in the video how lemon peels in the steam were providing the other woman with flu-like symptoms such unbelievable relief! Is that worth investigating? You bet! Here's what I found and what you need to know. In the July 2014 issue of *BioMed Research International*, Pantsulaia and colleagues found that lemon peel extract had decreased the levels of tumor necrosis factor (TNF-alpha) and interferon in patients with autoimmune hepatitis. Citrus peel extract has not only anti-inflammatory effects but anti-cancer effects also. Citrus peel is rich in two groups of chemicals that are responsible for its anti-inflammatory and anticancer effects, flavonones, and polymethoxylated flavanones PMF's). Interestingly, these two chemical compounds are rarely found in other plants and have anti-inflammatory, anticancer, antioxidant, and analgesic effects. In 2005, Kim et al showed that citrus extract causes stomach cancer cells to die. Citrus fruits such as oranges and grapefruits should therefore be required in our daily dietary recommendations. When you start feeling sick, advance to adding lemon peels to your diet. It just might save your life.

REMEDY 8

PRAYER TO GOD!

Genuine prayer is heartfelt prayer that moves the hand and heart of God. Pray for strength, forgiveness of your sins, healing, and for protection. Pray for your family, friends, neighbors, co-workers, employees, business partners, leaders and healthcare workers and the police.

Prayer works but don't subject yourself to liars and religious charlatans. Many of those that died of Covid-19 died alone without a priest, prophet, partner or parent at their bedside. EVEN PREACHERS WITH INTEGRITY HAVE DIED OF COVID. If they did not have God in their hearts and lives, imagine how terrible and lonely their last days on earth must have been. So make sure you have a genuine relationship with the God of heaven. Stop relying on religious rituals or your religious groups for your spiritual nourishment or direction. Talk to God as a person and get a Bible and read it. I have personally read the Bible over thirty-five times and I can assure you some of the statements in it will blow your mind as to its accuracy. That Bible will enable you to understand how to forge a relationship with God, one that you will truly need if you've been diagnosed with Covid-19. Remember the Prime Minister of Italy saying, they had done everything, and nothing worked but perhaps only God can.

Did you know the Bible, the spiritual guide to intimacy with God, says don't eat bats? Bats are the presumed primary host of the SARS-2 Corona virus that led to the Covid-19 pandemic. If there is a God, you bet he is much smarter than we humans. It would be wise to follow his advice than to argue. Here are the Bible verses:

13. *And these are they which ye shall have in abomination among the fowls; they shall not be eaten, they are an abomination: the eagle, and the ossifrage, and the ospray.*
14. *And the vulture and the kite after his kind;*
15. *Every raven after his kind;*
16. *And the owl, and the night hawk, and the cuckoo, and the hawk after his kind,*
17. *And the little owl, and the cormorant, and the great owl,*
18. *And the swan, and the pelican, and the gier eagle,*
19. *And the stork, the heron after her kind, and the lapwing, and the **bat**. Leviticus 11:13-19*

Notice that this list ends with one specific animal, the bat. It is clear God doesn't want us eating bats and the instruction was laid down 3500 years ago. We may not fully understand the reasons for the rule but we ought to trust and obey. If God created these animals, he also knows the microorganisms in them that may be harmful to us. If we choose, we might investigate but not through rebellion, aka bat soup! Our job is to obey even as we investigate. What we often do instead is disobey and then try to investigate, control and limit the consequences of our disobedience. Bats carry diseases that could be deadly to humans. You know of at least two, rabies and now SARS-CoV-1 and probably SARS-CoV-2. The Bible does not say

"thou shalt have Covid-19 if thou eat bats,"

Yet it's clear that the Bible seems to understand this possibility. Now we have a pandemic and corrupt scientists and frustrated doctors and patients. We not only eat and transfer zoonotic microorganisms that should have stayed in their own neighborhood on these animals, we even went digging through their feces looking for viruses! (*Shi Zhengli, 2013*). A zoonotic disease is an infectious disease that is transmitted between two species, from animals to humans or from humans to animals. Examples include anthrax, animal flu, bird flu, monkey pox and now, SARS-CoV-2. Intelligently ignore the controversy about the Wuhan lab leak. There really is no controversy about it. If you read page 41 of *Covid-19: Physician Treatment Strategies* (available at smashword.com) published in May 2020, you can tell the likely origin of SARS-CoV-2.

Prayer and meditation can ease the stress placed on your nervous and hormonal systems. Prayer and a strong confidence, faith and hope can replace your fear if you can learn to trust God. When things seem hopeless, you'll need to believe in something or someone bigger than yourself or your circumstances. God will do for most people. You have to decide what can calm your nerves and eliminate the fear and pain. Drugs will numb but not eliminate. Stress and fear can activate your immune and neurological systems, raise your blood pressure, heart rate, and reduce your ability to metabolize food and fat. This can lead to weight gain, hypertension, high cholesterol and arthritis. Stress and fear can also lead to irrational behaviors and group thinking.

Couples who find themselves stuck with each other at home must learn to be more caring, loving, patient and tolerate of each other. If you married someone for their money and were happy they were gone all the time, Covid-19 has brought them back home with love. You should wake up and start living in the real world. Get used to having your spouse around and build the skills for living with another human being who may in fact love you more than you can ever know. Pray together. Forgive. Touch and hold each other at least 5 times a day. Find a hobby. Buy sketchpads and get some drawing or painting instructions from YouTube. You might discover some fantastic talent you never knew you had. Master or upgrade your current skills. Find some seclusion time where you can reconnect your spirit soul and body in a quiet private place. Silence, not noise, is the great rejuvenator.

If you're facing death threats from Covid-19 or any other illness, then realize the truth about life, that it's a journey. No one is promised an extra day. Make every breath count. Live your life on purpose every day, every hour and every minute. If you've ever heard me speak about time, I look at life through seconds not minutes. So live life to the second and don't wait for the minute. Then pray,

God in heaven, if you are there, if you are real, help me. If it's true that sinners who ignore Jesus end up in hell, then forgive me of all my sins. I ask for Jesus to come into my heart today. Cleanse my heart of evil, and give me your eternal life and Holy Spirit. Heal me, comfort me, strengthen my family and I, and meet me right here where I am. I ask in Jesus' name. Amen.

Covid-19 creates a terror in the heart, causing men's hearts to fail for fear. You need something supernatural and divine to combat the uncertainty and fear. God and prayer can help you deal with your fear. Find a Christian group online if you can't find a good church. Read your Bible prayerfully. Listen to YouTube messages on holiness and purity. I also recommend the following on YouTube; Apostle Joshua Selman, Chuck Misler, Derek Prince, The Lion of Judah and Bishop TD Jakes. Spiritually elevating and calling music can be very helpful in calming your soul and reviving your spirit. I recommend Paul Wilbur's *For Your Name is Holy*. It's my number one favorite worship music. You might find something more suitable. The calmer the music and the less nerve jarring the instruments and vocals, the better it'll be for your soul.

REMEDY 9

HYDROGEN PEROXIDE (H2O2)

Spraying hydrogen peroxide into your nostrils immediately following exposure to Covid-19 patients could significantly reduce the impact of the exposure by denaturing the virus and its genetic material. Have a bottle of hydrogen peroxide in a small spray bottle container that does not allow light to penetrate through it. Hydrogen peroxide will otherwise degrade into oxygen and water and the peroxide effect neutralized completely if exposed to light. You spray it just as you would a saline spray, without inhaling or choking. A paramedic that transports a lot of Covid-19 patients to and from our emergency room once told me he uses food grade hydrogen peroxide. It's a little more expensive than the one you find over the counter. H2O2 is an additional remedy that can be protective against Covid-19 following exposure to high-risk individuals.

You may find conflicting evidence for or against the use of hydrogen peroxide or any of the other agents mentioned in this book as potential Covid-19 remedies. For example while it is clear that the bactericidal and virucidal effects of hydrogen peroxide can be applied to Covid-19 patients, *The Journal of Hospital Infection* published a review in October 11, 2020 *(Ortega et al., J Hosp Infect. Vol 106(4): 657-662)* stating that their systematic review of over one thousand articles revealed little scientific evidence of the effectiveness of virucidal activity of hydrogen peroxide. This article scores poorly on my criteria for judging clinical research papers published to help consumers and clinicians during this pandemic. The authors acted as if doing everything you can to prevent and curtail Covid-

19 is a game of intellect, as if lives are not at stake. Or perhaps, they do know lives are at stake and do not really care about those who may die from their disinformation tactics. Papers like this create a subtle impression that people should not use hydrogen peroxide as mouthwash. They expect you to remain neutral or passive when exposed to Covid-19, which in itself is a dangerous position that I completely disagree with. The paper meets some form of disinformation tactics that have been used to ensure that people continue to get infected with SARS-CoV-2 far longer than necessary. Besides the low utility score for the pandemic I gave this particular paper, you need to make sure that if something is safe, inexpensive, and has the possibility of being effective in helping you prevent Covid-19 infection, then use it if there are no contraindications. You can make sure that if anything goes wrong, you can get immediate medical attention. Most doctors at this point still won't treat you at the early stages with any known agent due to the same misinformation. Sadly, that means you're on your own. I once heard an anesthesiologist state that you as the patient is the one that has to make the decision that doctors ought to be making for you regarding treatment strategies for Covid-19. Annoying, but it's the cold hard truth resulting from intentional disinformation by multiple entities that stand to profit from the pandemic. Some academic centers and even reputable scientists have done an awful disservice to the entire global community through this disinformation. If something "may" be helpful, why on earth would you publish a paper that takes hours to put together, just to tell the world it "may" not work? Whenever you see an article or news item offering no practical solutions to fighting Covid-19 yet discourages any proactive measures ordinary people are trying to execute, be suspect of such an article, especially if the action you would have was safe, inexpensive, and easy to execute.

GARGLE Study Not Yet Studied!

There are few clinical trials that show us how much inertia exists amongst those providing scientific data on potential remedies in Covid-19. The GARGLE (Gargling Agents in Reducing Intraoral Viral Load Among Covid-19 Patients) is one of them. This GARGLE study registered with the ClinicalTrials.gov (Identifier NCT04341688) and posted on April 10, 2020 still has not started recruiting subjects as of January 13, 2021. Its estimated completion date is June 30, 2021. They've also estimated recruiting only 50 patients! The non-recruitment till now in June shows you their level of excitement. The bias in their choice of only 50 participants may not be readily appreciated since it is called a pilot study. The relative ease in performing this study should however have been a motivating factor to recruit far more patients if the goal was to find a simple, cost-effective, readily available solution to Covid-19. The number they intend to recruit is far too small. Even if the results turn out to be in favor of using mouthwashes in Covid-19 patients, the researchers can still misinform us by telling us they could not draw any reasonable conclusions from the study due to the small numbers. In effect the GARGLE study was set up to fail even before it is executed at this stage of the pandemic. That's how the influential *Covid-19 Industrial Complex* works.

REMEDY 10

FAMOTIDINE (Pepcid®)

Famotidine (Pepcid®) is an over the counter H2 antagonist useful in peptic ulcer prophylaxis and treatment and gastro-esophageal reflux patients. I would have placed this drug in the *Covid-19 Physician Treatment Strategies* book and not this book. I'm however not yet ready to update this book Information on useful Covid-19 remedies has been denied to both doctors and the lay population that need it the most. That's why I am including famotidine and its other counterpart, another antihistamine available over the counter, as remedies. In a few studies of hospitalized Covid-19 patients, famotidine, was found to be effective on multiple endpoints in Covid-19 patients when given alone or with the antihistamine cetirizine (Zyrtec®). You should contact your physician immediately following or suspected exposure to Covid-19 patients domestically or professionally. However since time is always of the essence following such exposure, you can immediately take over the counter medications that have been demonstrated to be helpful.

Dr. Hogan and colleagues reported their use of famotidine and cetirizine in Covid-19 patients with severe and critical respiratory symptoms. In this Mississippi study described in the August 29, 2020 issue of the journal, *Pulmonary Pharmacology & Therapeutics*, 110 patients between the ages of 17 and 97, (59.1% African American, 36.4% White, 4.5% other) received oral or intravenous cetirizine and famotidine for a minimum of 48 hours. The doses were famotidine 20mg and cetirizine 10mg administered in the emergency room or immediately on arrival to the Covid-19 unit. The combination of both drugs was continued every twelve hours and patients received a total of 4 doses. These patients had an average of 2.7 comorbidities; 78.2% had hypertension, 42.7% diabetes, 41.8% obesity, 26.4% had cardiac disease, 20% were smokers and 16.4% had morbid obesity and 10.9% had asthma. The intubation rate (*placing a life support breathing tube down the airway*) in the 110 patients admitted and treated with both drugs for a minimum of 48 hours was 7.3% and 93 patients (84.5%) were discharged. In spite of their higher comorbidities, the patients that received famotidine and cetirizine had far better outcomes than would have been ordinarily expected. Additional studies on the use of famotidine in Covid-19 patients have been reported by *Mather J.F et al, Am J Gastroenterology, 2020* and by *Freedberg et al., 2020*. During a pandemic, both drugs may help alleviate the burden created by Covid-19 infection on the healthcare system. Inflammatory cytokines are the pathway through which Covid-19 kills. Doing everything you can to block these mechanisms can save one life or many! So far, you'll only find some American doctors vehemently arguing against the use of early treatments. From what some of my colleagues and classmates outside the United States have expressed to me, these US doctors are probably the laughing stock of the rest of the physician world.

If anyone, particularly a doctor, tells you that a drug or treatment for Covid-19 can only be helpful if it is been tested in gold standard, randomized double-blinded placebo controlled trials, here are a few things you can tell them. First, what if enrolling patients to the placebo arm of such a clinical trial is unethical? Secondly, even if the drug were to be proven highly effective following randomized double blinded placebo controlled trials, is it the clinical trial that has conferred on the drug the ability to treat the condition? Didn't the drug have the property for managing the condition before the trial?

Or was it the trial that now conferred healing properties on the drug? ?

Thirdly, ask the doctor if he knows about the "Sackett" rule:

"The only way to be confident that a treatment is efficacious in the absence of randomized controlled trials is when traditional therapy is invariably followed by death."
- Sackett DL, Haynes RB, Guyatt GH, Tugwell P. Clinical Epidemiology: A Basic Science for Clinical Medicine. 1991.

As mentioned in *Covid-19 Physician Treatment Strategies*, the rule is called the Sackett-Haynes-Guyatt-Tugwell rule, and the short form name is "Sackett" rule. The rule is needed in this highly politicized and "divide and conquer" atmosphere that enriches Big Pharma but hurts patients, families and the economy. When you can't find randomized placebo controlled trials, it is not the end of evidence or the end of the world. It simply means the clinician has to do more mental work to arrive at what is best for patients. And if certain doctors are using their credentials to publish fallacious intellectual graffiti, then a clinician now has even more mental work to do. But that's exactly why we're doctors. We can do just that. If you find a doctor who cannot understand why you are skeptic about the vaccines, you've found one that cannot or refuses to do the necessary mental work or critical thinking.

Lastly, the scientific publishing world depends on advertising dollars from vaccine and drug manufacturers. Major scientific journals that have a physician readership are therefore unlikely to publish studies on inexpensive early treatments that will properly inform doctors on safe early treatments. Publishing inexpensive early treatments will hurt their number one customer and their biggest source of revenue, Big Pharma. According to Scott Neslin, a marketing professor, for every dollar spent, the return to drug advertisers averages about $5. So for the $448 million spent by drug companies advertising in medical journals in 2003, the return would be roughly over $2 billion. The big nine multispecialty journals we read are *NEJM, JAMA, Annals, Lancet, BMJ, Canadian Medical Journal, American Family Physician, Medical Journal of Australia* and *PLoS Medicine. PLoS Medicine* is the only one that does not accept advertisements for drugs or medical devices. Hopefully, you can see why information on early treatments is not finding it easy to get to the public domain. The major sponsors of clinical trials are the same ones that benefit the most from vaccines. Why should we expect them to sponsor or pay for research that attacks their profits? If some doctors finally fund their own research and send it to the same major scientific and medical journals, the editors will find enough reasons to reject the papers.

If the major journals accept and publish the results of well-executed clinical trials on inexpensive treatments, Big Pharma may punish them by cutting their advertising budgets to that particular journal. These journals will therefore not publish the results of successful inexpensive treatments. They will however gladly publish failed inexpensive trials, as well as *randomized control tricks* and questionably fabricated papers like the ones retracted from the May 2020 Lancet and New England journals on the "dangerous drug" hydroxychloroquine.

The depth of this entanglement between scientific journals and the drug companies is very difficult to disrupt as money, lots of it, is involved even before the pandemic. Both entities mutually benefit from the relationship and it is a very profitable one. This relationship has been partly responsible for the relative lack of information on early treatments for Covid-19 and may partly explain the persistence of the pandemic to date. This kind of entanglement is why medical students, residents and fellows are informed of the need to critically assess the literature. You don't need to learn how to critically assess the obituary column of any newspaper. If you see a picture of someone who died in the obituary section of a local newspaper, that person in almost all likelihood is dead. No need to sit down wit a gallon of coffee to critically analyze the write up in order to figure out if the person is really dead. Yet when "trusted scientists" publish a clinical trial, we must critically analyze the paper to see whether there is a lie or if it's all the truth. Every doctor knows that's the norm. But what does this norm imply in the real world? That these "trusted scientists" publishing in a reputable journal may not be telling the whole truth! I'm sure they have enough brains to see the entire picture of the truth in their own study. Yet the paper can still lie! The reason for the partial truth or lies is simply driven by pharmaceutical companies. This is how far those lies have now brought us. According to a paper by Dr. Lisa Schwartz, MD and Steven Woloshin, MD, *(JAMA. 2019;321(1):80-96),* direct to consumer prescription drug advertising rose from $1.3 billion in 1997 to $6 billion in 2016 with "a shift towards advertising high-cost biologics and cancer immunotherapies. Marketing to healthcare professionals was highest, going from $15.6 billion to $20.3 billion during the same period. The tobacco industry bought advertising space from JAMA at a time when the journal was struggling financially and became its biggest advertiser. It's time for the medical community to change the criteria for publishing and rejecting clinically relevant scientific papers. The amount and type of advertising allowed in medical journals needs revision too.

REMEDY 11

CETIRIZINE

Cetirizine is an antihistamine sold over the counter. It is indicated for the treatment of allergic rhinitis, seasonal allergies and chronic urticaria. It was used successfully alongside famotidine in Covid-19 patients in some clinical trials as stated in the last chapter. It was given as 10mg every 12 hours for a total of 4 doses. Doctors outside the United States have been using this drug for sometime in their Covid-19 patients. It's use in allergies and inflammatory-type reactions may theoretically make it an effective agent in Covid-19 patients. In real clinical situations, cetirizine in combination with Famotidine showed significant clinical impact in Covid-19 patients as you saw in the previous chapter. The WHO physician who heads over 10,000 doctors that spoke with me said they also use cyproheptadine in Covid-19 patients. Antihistamines may play an important role in reducing the negative impact of the burden of disease created by Covid-19. The mechanisms may not be clear but cetirizine should be considered an important remedy following suspected exposure to Covid-19. *(Blanco J et al., Pulmonary Pharmacology & Therapeutics. 2021 April. 67:101989)* Make sure you see your doctor before taking any of these medications. Cetirizine has anti-inflammatory properties. It has also been shown to reduce cytokines in children with perennial allergic rhinitis. *(Ciprandi et al., Eur Ann Allergy Clin Immunol. 2004 Jun;36(6): 237-240).*

REMEDY 12

GARLIC

Garlic (*Allium sativum L.*) has a long-standing history as a medicinal bulbous plant with multiple uses for centuries. It is used in different cultures around the world. Its main active compound allicin is formed when intact garlic-containing alliin is chopped and the enzyme alliinase is activated. Not only does garlic lower serum cholesterol, and blood pressure (*Ried et al., 2013a; Stabler et al., 2012; Auer et al., 1990*), it also inhibits platelet aggregation. (*Chen et al., 2013*). Inhibition of platelet aggregation reduces the likelihood of coronary thromboses otherwise known as a heart attack. Not only does garlic reduce the growth rate of cancer cells, it may be the most potent food with cancer prevention properties (*Kweon et al., 2003; Amagase & Milner, 1993; Hsing et al., 2002*) according to the US National Cancer Institute. (*Dahanukar & Thatte, 1997*). The claims of garlic as an antiviral are limited in terms of high quality clinical trial data. Nevertheless, its use as an antiviral remedy is without question. Its safety in pregnancy, breastfeeding and young children is unclear. A review on garlic published by Leyla Bayan et al., (*Ayurveda Journal of Phytomedicine (AJP), Vol 4, No.1 Jan-Feb 2014*), might be worth reading. Researchers at the Iranian Pasteur Institute published an interesting article demonstrating potent antiviral effects of garlic on Influenza A. (*Mehrbod et al., Iranian Journal of Virology 2009;3(1):19-23*). The other active ingredients in garlic that make it a potential agent in this pandemic include sulfur-containing phytochemicals such ajoenes (E and Z) and diallyl sulfide. (*Sucheta et al., 2020; Razina et al., 2020*). Molecular docking analysis shows alliin has high antiviral activity that could potentially prevent Covid-19, particularly in combination with other potentially useful remedies mentioned in this book or elsewhere. *(Rajagopal et al, 2020; Pandey et al 2021).*

Eat your garlic and add it generously to your foods. If you get sick or suspect Covid-19 exposure, see your healthcare provider immediately.

REMEDY 13

TURMERIC

Turmeric (Curcuma longa) is a potent medicinal plant. Turmeric's main active ingredient is curcumin. Curcumin has been shown to have antioxidant, anti-inflammatory, anti-diabetic and anti-cancer properties. *(Zhang D et al., Evid Based Complement Alternat Med. 2013 Nov 24.)* It also has a very low toxicity. It has also been shown to reduce the development of Alzheimer's disease. *(Hishikawa et al., Ayu. 2012 Oct-Dec;33(4):499-504)* This pandemic has led some medical writers to come up with conflicting messages regarding turmeric, rather than outline and emphasize its benefits. You won't find this surprising if you've read chapter 10. That's however unfair to the average consumer. Nevertheless, here is one major article showing that curcumin, an active ingredient of turmeric, reduces the concentration of tumor necrosis factor TNF-α. TNF-α is one of the inflammatory cytokines that lead to the multiple complications associated with Covid-19 infection. Published in 2016, and therefore quite reliable than many of the more recently published 2020 articles during the pandemic denouncing turmeric or curcumin. This article by Amirhossein et al., *(Pharmacol Res. May 2016)* is a systematic review of 8 randomized control trials showing that curcumin was effective in reducing TNF-α and in reducing circulating levels of another inflammatory cytokine, IL-6. *(Giuseppe et al, Pharmacol Res. 2016 Sep.)*

Curcumin has been shown to inhibit angiotensin 2-induced inflammation of rat vascular smooth muscle *(Li, et al, Int J Mol Med. 2017; 39(5):1307-1316)* as well as reducing the angiotensin-2 induced myocardial fibrosis in rats. *(Pang et al, Drug Des Devel Ther. 2015;9:6043-6054)*. Not too surprisingly, an article appeared in nutraingredients.com by Will Chu on April 20, 2020 at 13:06 GMT stating that French authorities (ANSES, Agency for Food, Environmental and Occupational Health & Safety) are warning of turmeric-containing food supplements interfering with inflammatory defense mechanisms that fight the coronavirus. You can see what planet they live on! To think they said this the same month the first edition of this book came out means they had the right information but were not capable of disseminating what was needed to the populace. Curcumin can block entry of the virus, asides from its beneficial anti-inflammatory and antioxidant effects. Did ANSES get it wrong! There are still credible scientific articles written during the pandemic that demonstrate the potential benefits of curcumin in helping curb the pandemic. One of such articles is a 2020 review article by Nanchang University's Ziteng Liu and Professor Ying Ying. (*The Inhibitory effect of Curcumin on Virus-Induced Cytokine Storm and its Potential Use in the Associated Severe Pneumonia. Cell Dev Biol., 12 June 2020*). Take your turmeric in moderate doses and if you suspect you have Covid-19, see your healthcare provider immediately.

REMEDY 14

BROMHEXINE

Bromhexine hydrochloride (BH) is an alkaloid obtained from the plant *Justicia adhatoda*. It is used in cough mixtures and has been shown to prevent SARS-CoV-2 invading our cells. Bromhexine hydrochloride stimulates the activity of the ciliated epithelium, triggering the hydrolysis of mucus proteins. It increases lysosomal activity and is metabolized to several compounds that include ambroxol, a known mucolytic. Bromhexine hydrochloride inhibits the entry of SARS-CoV-2 into the lung cells by blocking an enzyme (TMPRSS2) the virus uses to gain entry into the target cells. This enzyme activates the S1 subunit of the spike protein so it can then attach to the ACE-2 receptor on the outer surface of the special lung cell called a type-II pneumocyte. Once it attaches to the ACE-2 receptor of the type II pneumocyte, the next step for the virus is to get inside the lung cell. Blocking the enzyme TMPRSS2 with bromhexine could therefore potentially prevent infection with Covid-19.

In a randomized open label clinical trial of 78 patients, 8mg three times daily of bromhexine hydrochloride was given to Covid-19 patients. *(Ansarin et al., Bioimpacts 2020; 10(4): 209-215)*. Those that received BH had significantly reduced intensive care unit (ICU) admissions (2/39 vs. 11/39, p=0.006), reduced intubations (1/39 vs. 9/39, p= 0.007) and reduced deaths (0 vs. 5, p=0.027). According to the paper, early administration of oral bromhexine hydrochloride is a safe and effective treatment for patients with Covid-19. It is an old over the counter medication. This paper was published in July 2020 but has never been mentioned by the health authorities. Another 2020 article published by Drs. Dmitry Stepanov & Peter Lierz in the open access *J Infect Dis Epidemiol 6:135.doi.org/10.23937)* recommended that BH be started as soon as a patient shows symptoms, early in the course of Covid-19 infection.

If you suspect you have Covid-19, see your doctor immediately.

REMEDY 15

POVIDONE IODINE

Povidone-iodine (Betadine®, PVP-I) is an antiseptic frequently used in many US hospitals and clinics. It has a very broad antiseptic spectrum and high virucidal activity. It was shown to effectively inactivate SARS-CoV-1 in vitro as a 0.23 -1% solution as far back as 2006. (*Kawira et al., 2006*). In a study reported in the *June 7, 2018* issue of the *Infectious Disease Therapy* journal, Dr. Eggers and colleagues also reported rapid bactericidal activity using a 7% PVP-I solution. In the same study, a 0.23% PVP-I solution, when used as a gargle or mouthwash, rapidly inactivated SARS-CoV-1, Middle East Respiratory Syndrome-related coronavirus (MERS-CoV) as well as H1N1 influenza virus following 15 seconds of exposure to the PVP-I solution. How much inactivation? Close to 100%!

Three years earlier, in the *September 28, 2015* issue of the *Infectious Disease Therapy* journal, Dr. Eggers and colleagues had reported a 99.99% reduction in the viral load of MERS-CoV in the mouth and pharynx of infected subjects following application of a 1% PVP-I solution used as a gargle or mouthwash. In another study reported in the October 27, 2020 issue of the *Journal of Otolaryngology - Head and Neck Surgery,*Dr. Syed Naqvi and colleagues used the following protocol:

> *For pre-induction of anesthesia, 15ml of 1% PVP-I was used as swish for 30 seconds and spit and 10-20 ml of 1% PVP-I the solution was applied to the nasal cavity for 30 seconds.*

PVP-I solutions have been shown to reduce absenteeism due to common cold and influenza in middle school children. *(Shiraishi & Nakagawa, 2002)*. While common cold and influenza are viral infections, the PVP-I solution in this study was also shown to simultaneously cause a 99.4% reduction in bacterial count. There is ample evidence for judicious use of povidone iodine in prevention of SARS-CoV-2 infection as a gargle and mouthwash and perhaps swabbing in the nostrils following high-risk exposure to a Covid-19 patient.

REMEDY 16

ZINC

Zinc is a trace element and since the pandemic, virtually everyone around the world now takes it regularly. The zinc sold in most pharmacies is zinc sulfate 220mg and contains 50mg of elemental zinc. Typical dosing is 50mg daily when using early treatment regimens. The recommended daily allowance of zinc is 11mg for males and 8mg for females. *(Katz, Friedman & Lucan. Nutrition in Clinical Practice. 2015).* Zinc is an important trace element necessary for growth, reproductive health, immune function, smell and taste. It is involved in hundreds of enzymatic processes in the body. Zinc deficiency can present as infertility, recurrent viral infections, growth retardation in children, skin problems night blindness, hair loss, and loss of smell and taste. Zinc affects DNA and RNA synthesis. Zinc is a catalyst in almost 2000 enzymatic processes in the body. *(Read SA et al., The Role of Zinc in Antiviral Immunity. Advances in Nutrition. 10 (4):696-710. July 2019).*

What does zinc really do as a potential remedy in Covid-19? It has broad-spectrum antiviral activity and specifically inhibits the activity of a particular enzyme, *RNA dependent RNA polymerase (RdRp).*

> *"RdRp is the same enzyme that allows SARS-CoV-2 to use your protein synthesis factory inside your cells to produce more coronavirus particles. How quickly would you want to block this process?"- The HCQ Debate, p 151*

As far back as 2010, increased intracellular concentrations of zinc were shown to inhibit replication (multiplication) of SARS-CoV-1 in vitro and in cell cultures. *(Aartwan JW et al., PLoS Pathogens. November 4, 2010)*. When agents called ionophores such as pyrithione are added to these in vitro solutions and cell cultures, much lower concentrations of zinc are required to inhibit the virus. Ionophores are chemicals that allow zinc to enter easily into the cells and allow higher concentrations of zinc to build up inside the cell. Naturally, zinc has some challenge crossing the cell membrane but that difficulty is reduced by ionophores like hydroxychloroquine and quercetin. Several studies have demonstrated the ability of these zinc-zinc ionophore (z-zi) combinations to inhibit multiple viruses including rhinoviruses that cause the common cold *(Gaudernak et al.,. J Virol 76:6004-6015)*, and the foot and mouth virus infection *(Polatnick & Bachrach. Antimicrob Agents Chemotherap. 13:731-734)*. Zinc also prevented hepatitis E replication in vitro by blocking the *RdRp* enzyme.

Zinc had also shown promise in inhibiting HIV-1 replication as far back as 1991. *(Zhang et al., 1991)*. Years later, in 1999, another group of scientists showed that zinc inhibits HIV-1 viral transcription. *(Haraguchi et al., Antiviral Res. 1999; 43(2): 123-133)*. Zinc has also been shown to be effective in inhibiting herpes simplex virus types 1 and 2 as well as hepatitis E virus. *(Kaushik N et al., J Virol. 91(21). November 2017)*.

Even viral warts clear after zinc was used in the treatment of recalcitrant warts in two randomized placebo controlled trials. *(Al-Gurairi et al., Br J Dermatol. 2002;146(3): 423-431; Yagboobi et al., J Am Acad Dermatol. 2009;60(4):70-708)*. The greatest responses of viral warts to oral zinc were in zinc-deficient patients. A high incidence of zinc deficiency or lower levels of zinc was noted in patients with persistent viral warts. *(Raza et al., J Coll Physicians Surg Pak. 2010;20(2):83-6)*.

There are more than 30 human proteins responsible for zinc balance (homoeostasis) in order to prevent zinc toxicity. Excess zinc or zinc toxicity can still occur and lead to copper deficiency. Copper deficiency can manifest as skin and hair abnormalities, low blood counts and bone loss.

Zinc has also been shown to inhibit several other viruses including the picorna viruses *(Lanke et al., J Gen Virol 8:1206-1217)*, Coxackie virus *(Si X et al., J Virol 79: 8014-8023)* and human papilloma virus *(Kim JH et al., Gynecol Oncol. 2011;122(2):303-306.*

Viruses and cancer are two of man's greatest medical challenges even in the twenty-first century. Yet zinc seems to have an uncanny ability to hinder the replication of several viruses. Is the entire world unconsciously improving its own overall health without realizing it by ingesting zinc? The chances are quite high that if we are able to supplement our diet with enough zinc we might accomplish more for our health than we can imagine. Since every adversity has a seed of an equivalent or greater blessing *(Napoleon Hill, Think and Grow Rich. 1937)*, our increased intake of zinc might be Covid-19's long-term blessing in disguise against many viral infections, despite the well-known tragedies it has brought into our lives and countries.

REMEDY 17

QUERCETIN

Quercetin is a flavonol. Flavonols belong to the flavonoids, naturally occurring anti-oxidants that include flavones, flavonols and isoflavones. Flavones are present in citrus fruits, while soybeans contain significant amounts of isoflavones. *(Katz, Friedman & Lucan, Nutrition in Clinical Practice. 3rd Ed. 2015).* Flavonoids are also found in grapes, nuts, cocoa and dark chocolate. Flavonoid-rich dark chocolate has been shown to improve platelet function in smokers *(Herman et al., Heart 2006;92:119-120).*

What does all this have to do with Covid-19? Quercetin is not just an antioxidant it is also a zinc ionophore. It allows high concentrations of zinc to form inside the cells. As you know when zinc is inside the cells, it can inhibit RdRp thereby preventing SARS-CoV-2 from replication inside the infected cell. The paper, *Synergistic Effect of Quercetin and Vitamin C Against COVID-19,* is still awaiting publication more than seven months after it was submitted for publication in November 16, 2020. In this study of quercetin and vitamin C in healthcare workers (HCW) with a high exposure to Covid-19, 71 patients received 500mg quercetin daily, 500 vitamin C daily, and 50mg bromelain daily (QCB) in two divided doses. The control group consisted of 42 HCW subjects with similarly high risk for Covid-19 exposure. These 42 subjects did not receive any supplements. Subjects were followed for 120 days and the final point of the study was either termination of QCB use or detection of coronavirus infection. There were no significant differences between the two groups except for age: the QCB group was about 6 years older (39.0+/-8.8 years) than the control group of 42 subjects (32.9+/-8.7 years). The average follow-up for the QCB group was 113 days and 118 days for the control group. During the follow up, 1 HCW in the QCB group and 9 in the control group developed Covid-19. The transmission risk hazard for those that did not get QCB was 12.04 (95% CI 1.26-115.06; p=0.03). This study showed that QCB administration was protective for healthcare workers. The details of the clinical trial registration are NCT04377789. The authors are *Arslan B, Ergun NU, Topuz S, Semerci SY, Suner N, Kocatas A & Onal H. The article is yet to be peer-approved.* I'm skeptic about when this paper will finally be published. Bromelain is a mixture of enzymes found in pineapple that help with protein digestion. It has anti-inflammatory as well as wound healing properties.

Quercetin has anti-inflammatory and anti-oxidant properties and is also a zinc ionophore. Given early in Covid-19 infection, it may help with combating viral replication as well as the inflammation. As an immune booster and nutritional supplement, quercetin can be taken at a dose of 250mg daily and increased to twice daily following Covid-19 infection based on your healthcare provider's recommendations. Be sure to inform your primary care doctor if you have to start any nutritional supplements mentioned in this book or elsewhere.

Quercetin can be mocked by those paid to misinform the pubic about any early treatments. If you cannot get a doctor to start you on early treatment following a diagnosis of Covid-19 infection, you ought to start taking this supplement with zinc in the recommended doses. Keep in mind that even beneficial medications or vitamins can become poisons when not used correctly.

Please read the disclaimer on page 4 of this book.

REMEDY 18

VITAMIN D

Vitamin D is a fat-soluble vitamin found in dairy, cod liver oil, salmon, fortified milk and tuna. Low levels of vitamin D have been associated with lower performance during pulmonary function testing in children. *(Alyasin S et al., Allergy Asthma Immuno Res 2011;3(4):251-255).* Vitamin D has been shown to inhibit pro-inflammatory cytokine production *(Zhang Y et al., J Immunol. 2012;188(5):2127-2135).* Vitamin D is involved in modulating the innate and acquired immunity, and the production of antimicrobial proteins such as cathelicidin and defensin. Vitamin D is also involved in the pathways that control the intracellular destruction of microorganisms at the genetic level. Normal vitamin D levels (25-OH) are necessary for a diverse range of functions including calcium metabolism, immune regulation and cancer prevention. Normal levels of vitamin D (25-OH) are 75nmol/L (30ng/mL). Vitamin D insufficiency refers to levels of 50-75nmol/L (20-29ng/mL and vitamin D deficiency is diagnosed when vitamin D levels are less than 50nmol/L (less than 20ng/mL).

In a British study of over 6000 adult patients, the incidence of vitamin D levels were shown to correlate with the incidence of influenza infection. The study *(Berry et al., Br. J Nutr. 2011, 106, 1433-1440)* showed that for every 10nmol/L rise in vitamin D levels, the incidence of respiratory tract infections decreased by 7%.

In another review of 18 prospective studies *(Ma Y et al., Am Soc Clin Oncol 2011:3775-3782),* a dose dependent protective effect of higher levels of vitamin D against colorectal cancer was found for each 10ng/mL increase in vitamin D levels. Several studies have shown that vitamin D plays a highly significant role as an anti-inflammatory agent. *(Yu et al. Proc. Natl. Acad. Sci. USA 1995, 92, 10990-10994).*

How much vitamin D should you take? It depends. 1000U is recommended by most as normal daily intake but you should talk to your doctor first. If you have kidney stones, taking large doses of vitamin D could send you into the emergency room more frequently with kidney stones or worse. You need to check regularly with your primary care provider when taking vitamin D supplements.

REMEDY 19:

Follow The Rules!

You should follow all the rules of quarantine, social isolation, personal hygiene, infection control, reporting, or any other recommendations intended to keep you and everyone else from spreading the virus or dying unnecessarily. Stay healthy and drop as much unnecessary weight as you possibly can. From the patients I have taken care of, Covid-19 hits the morbidly obese really hard. Always remember that 6 feet of social distancing is insufficient when you're not wearing protective gear during a pandemic. If someone sneezes nearby, subsequent airborne viruses could reach you at 27 feet. I explained the science behind this in the physician's version of this series, *COVID-19: Physician Treatment Strategies,* available at the publisher's website, smashword.com. It's a very detailed book on how Covid-19 should be diagnosed and managed effectively and how the disease results in death. I didn't want to waste any more time once Amazon tried to block the first edition of this book last year from reaching the public. I shared more details about this censorship in the latter part of this book.

Psychological stress from isolation demands that you learn techniques of emotional self-regulation. Mindfulness, meditation, reading, listening to god calming music, avoiding anger outbursts can all be helpful. Avoid toxic relationships and hostile interactions with others. Respect your life and that of others around you. Don't rebel against rules you know are designed to protect you and others if adhered to. If someone sneezes in your face and the vaccine doesn't protect you, would a facemask at least have provided some barrier to reducing the viral load inhaled? Do you realize that even in most hospitals treating Covid-19 patients, the nurses and staff routinely wear surgical masks to protect themselves? If you come in contact with a person you suspect has Covid-19 and inhaled the same air they exhaled, don't panic. Use the remedies described in this book.

Continued lockdowns have been questioned and mandatory vaccinations are indicators of political power craze and scientific tyranny of a few obnoxious group.

REMEDY 20

Rest & Relax

You must get enough rest and sleep. Working 7 days non-stop, particularly in a demanding job can burn down your immune system. You could burnout not just mentally, emotionally and physically, but immunologically and spiritually. Just one night of 4 hours of sleep deprivation can increase the production of cytokines in your body. Such sleep deprivation can increase tumor necrosis factor (TNF-α) and Interleukin-6 (IL-6). *(Irwin et al, 2008)* These are dangerous chemicals that are partly responsible for the cytokine storm that eventually kills most Covid-19 patients.

Similarly, sleep deprived married couples had higher levels of (TNF-α) and Interleukin-6 (IL-6) after discussing a marital problem. *(Kiecolt-Glaser et al., Psychoneuroendocrinology. May 2017)*.

Get enough sleep. Enjoy your life. Find and do something you love. Create a bucket list. Find time to laugh. Spend time with your loved ones. Change your philosophy about life and find reasons to always be grateful. Learn to keep your mind still even if you have to retrain it through active memorization. *(Bible Vitamins: Neuroplasticity and The Untapped Power of Bible Verses 2018)*. Learn to practice mindfulness even if you don't want to engage in meditation.

While adequate sleep boosts your immune system and calms you nervous system, anxiety wreaks havoc on both!

Chapter 21

Dr. USA: No Treatment for Covid-19?

While some doctors and healthcare practitioners took a stand to prescribe hydroxychloroquine (HCQ) and other agents as part of their early treatment regimen for Covid-19 patients, the US Government agencies like the CDC, NIH, and FDA continued to avoid HCQ, Ivermectin or any other inexpensive and effective drugs for early treatment. Some doctors, seemingly overwhelmed by the amount of anecdotal and scientific evidence chose to play safe and would not prescribe either Ivermectin or HCQ. Many of these doctors and healthcare practitioners allowed patients that could have benefitted from such treatments to slip through their hands, and sadly, sometimes into the cold hands of death.

The drugs for early treatment are inexpensive, safe, and have been in use for decades for other indications. When the only other option seems to be death, what should a healthcare professional do? Go ahead and prescribe or just sit down and hope the patient gets better? The hope strategy, hoping the Covid-19 patient will not get worse or die seems to be a passive and dangerous approach considering the risk of death, particularly in high-risk patients. Such a hopeless finger-biting strategy is not only harmful it is also a reckless approach to a major killer pandemic. Such behavior contradicts the Hippocratic oath, and indicates some cognitive dissonance. Any physician playing safe while a patient's life is at stake is afraid of something and is surely not practicing medicine. A physician who does that knows that what he or she is doing is wrong. Wouldn't it have been better to prescribe a safe drug with a probability of a favorable outcome? Even if we don't have all the answers as to why or how the drug works, it's still better to treat early than to leave the patient at the mercy of death or disability. While theoretically, the possibility exists that the Covid-19 illness could be self-limiting, the reality of Covid-19 deaths demands that a doctor do something helpful to Covid-19 positive patients. Early treatments are relatively safe and the benefit-risk assessment highly favors their use. In addition the drugs are relatively inexpensive, available, with decades of safety data. Some pharmacies also refused to fill HCQ prescriptions. It was therefore hard to find a doctor in the United States treating early Covid-19, or mentioning the word "HCQ". You had to be a brave doctor to do all that. And a lo of people died because doctors feared attacks from multiple sources.

CNN's Elizabeth Cohen and another colleague reported on June 17, 2020 on cnn.com website that the US Stockpile was stuck with 63 million doses of unused hydroxychloroquine. No small thanks to medical journalism terrorists, as well as the NIH, CDC and FDA. Things could have been different if the deceased patients and current long haulers had received HCQ early in the course of their illness. A good percentage of the 600,000 plus dead patients in the US would probably would have survived and thrived! More than 10 million infected patients could have been treated early. On top of this, and with total disregard for pharmacologic and pathophysiologic principles, the FDA undermined physicians by knowingly recommending that we only prescribe HCQ at the late stages of illness, in hospitalized patients. This in itself is not only gross incompetence but may be considered an act of treason. The FDA stated clearly that HCQ should not be given when it would work best, in outpatient settings. They recommended we give it when it was most likely to fail. The FDA also added another hindrance. Outside the hospital, HCQ was to be used only in clinical trials. Yet the majority of early Covid-19 infected patients that needed early treatment had no access to such clinical trials or to doctors engaged in clinical trials. They only had access to treating doctors in regular clinics and emergency rooms. As explained in *The HCQ Debate*, even those patients with immediate access to clinical trials were not managed properly. Some didn't receive the drug within a reasonable time frame while others were given lethal doses of hydroxychloroquine. I explained this in greater detail in the book. In the end cognitive dissonance plagued well-meaning doctors once they saw the FDA EUA recommendations to use HCQ only in clinical trials or in hospitalized patients. This was a strategic move probably engineered behind the scenes by Big Pharma. Clearly, Big Pharma, not patients or the doctors treating them, benefits from such nonsense.

In the real world of Covid-19, with death and hospitalization and progressive worsening of symptoms even following hospitalization were inevitable. Tying the hands of doctors with regulations like the EUA limiting prescribing to hospitalized patients and clinical trials, was predictably going to cost many Americans their lives from Covid-19. There should be no doubt that even hesitating for some days could cost many patients their lives or livelihoods. Rather than act and prescribe, many doctors froze at the thought of prescribing these drugs. These are probably extremely busy doctors that paid far more attention to the news than to the detailed reading of their research journals or to their own intuitive sense. Many seemed overwhelmed by the opposing views been released by two groups: those in favor and those against a particular early treatment. As a result many did nothing. That was a problem. They abandoned the Hippocratic oath by passivity and many patients probably died as a result. "Do no harm" to these practitioners during the pandemic meant do nothing, even though doing nothing harmed the patient far more than prescribing safe drugs the media was now lying about. This freeze unfortunately has been partly responsible for the death of over half a million Americans. Contrast this with a coroner in one of the small cities in the United States. This man knew that the death toll in this small city would eventually fall on him. Fortunately, he was also a licensed doctor. Having his own private practice, he began to research and came across enough data to begin prescribing HCQ. He didn't wait for irrefutable evidence, much of which was been distorted or suppressed anyway. He just asked if there was enough evidence to warrant prescribing HCQ. The answer was a resounding yes. He also considered what precautions to take while prescribing HCQ to patients with heart disease after purchasing *The HCQ Debate: What Did Researchers Hide:*

> *After seeing his last patient for the day in his clinic last summer, Dr. CJ walked about 50 yards to the hospital emergency room. He asked the nurses how he could purchase the book, The HCQ Debate. They helped him download the Amazon app and ordered the book. Two days later, and convinced by the information in the book, he started prescribing HCQ to Covid-19 patients. I worked as an ER physician in the same hospital, seeing an average of 3 to 4 Covid-19 patients daily at varying stages of illness. We often transferred them by ambulance or flew them out by helicopter. Two months later, I saw only one patient in 48 hours. Curious about the sudden drop in Covid-19 patients visits to the ER, the nurses I asked said the coroner was partly responsible. Dr. CJ had been prescribing HCQ for every Covid-19 patient before they got really ill to require hospitalization.*

Why were there only few other doctors doing the same thing? Edmund Burke, the 18th century Irish politician said,

"No passion so effectually robs the mind of its powers of acting and reasoning as fear."

Fear! A physician friend and podcaster surveyed 35 experienced and actively practicing physicians in North Carolina. All of them understood the high likelihood that HCQ could help their Covid-19 patients. Yet not one of them prescribed it. "But why", my friend, Dr. Winn Henderson asked this doctors? They all replied they were scared someone might come after them. This is a behavior that without doubt has contributed to many unnecessary deaths from Covid-19 in the United States. Economist and Harvard psychiatrist, Dr. J. Niels Rosenquist explained this HCQ prescribing freeze amongst healthcare professionals in an article published in the January issue of the *New England Journal of Medicine*. He called the overall confusion amongst healthcare professionals regarding Covid-19 and its proper management based on the available evidence *Bayesian Fatigue*:

Bayesian Fatigue is

"A stress induced dysphoria that is experienced when the corpus of knowledge that one has acquired over years to decades and that is the foundation of one's work, becomes less important than information that's been gathered from disparate sources in real time."
— J. Niels Rosenquist. *N Eng J Med. January 7, 2021*

A simplification of Dr. Rosenquist's observation above is that doctors have become disheartened and perhaps disoriented from the absence of gold standard RCTs for treating Covid-19 patients. Rather than these gold standards, genuine and clinically significant results that cannot be ignored are showing up from unexpected sources and in unexpectedly high numbers. Yet no matter how many of such cases are reported, ther will always be a counter argument from some "reputable TV expert doctor." So many studies came out showing that doctors could use HCQ in early Covid-19. For example, the Italian retrospective CORIST study of 3,451 hospitalized patients *(Di Castelnuovo et al. Eur. J Intern Med. 2020)* showed a 30% reduction in mortality in HCQ treated patients. That's a lot of patients. A doctor in his right mind just cannot ignore such results even if the study is not a gold standard study. Another example is the observational report in Belgium of 8075 patients *(Catteau et al., Int J Antimicrobial Agents. Vol 56, Issue 4, October 2020)*. There were several others with loads of patients improving on HCQ but there arose an anti-HCQ movement for political reasons and for profit. Doctors have been trained to look for gold standard RCTs. Not having this became mentally tasking, particularly when added to the misinformation from the media and the censoring. What is this gold standard doctors are looking for?

The Gold Standard RCT
Researchers use a "Gold Standard" method for accurately studying and reporting the safety and effectiveness of a drug in clinical trials. This gold standard is a carefully designed prospective randomized placebo controlled double-blinded trial (RCT). It provides the most important information about the effectiveness and safety of a drug or vaccine. Whenever you have an RCT, practicing physicians can confidently and comfortably use the published results of the trial to manage their patients whenever applicable. You can therefore say that the "Gold Standard" clinical trial evidence creates a comfort zone for the doctor treating patients using the study data. When clinical trials less than the gold standard are the only ones available, it's not the end of the world. It just means a doctor now has to do more mental work by critically evaluating these other studies. Most of us are

too busy to find the time to do this. Others find this exciting, while others find it unnecessarily stressful.

Unfortunately, in the real world, a practicing doctor won't always have an RCT when making a decision to prescribe a drug for an illness or condition. They can however make informed logical treatment decisions. These will be based on options gleaned from the published research data, an understanding of the disease process, a method for properly evaluating the literature, to individualize the care of the patient based on their clinical experience and expertise. That's how Covid-19 and its treatment should have been addressed from the outset. Instead of making information available to doctors treating Covid-19 patients, contradictory information began to surface from the mainstream media regarding any useful treatments. At the same time, social media began censoring and blocking any other information sources that could contribute to a doctor's intelligent decision making process. Worse, journalists began attacking reputable physicians like Didier Raoult, Harvey Risch and entire institutions like Detroit's Henry Ford Healthcare system. While this was going on, ill-conceived clinical trials and occasionally outright fraudulent clinical trials were also been published. Most of them were directed against early treatment agents. In some of these clinical trials poisonous doses of treatment drugs were given to patients. The results were published as randomized control tricks in reputable journals. One such example of the latter was the Recovery Clinical trial in the UK. Research like the RECOVERY, (2020) Mitja et al., (2020) Bouleware et al, (2020) and Tang et al., (2020), made it extremely difficult for doctors to figure out what was best for Covid-19 patients seen in the outpatient settings. There was little direction from the CDC or NIH.

Pfizer's Cure and Pirbright Institute's Coronavirus

Pfizer, the first company to manufacture the mRNA vaccine, went into the manufacturing phase of their vaccine on January 10, 2020 only nine days after news broke out from China about SARS-CoV-2 pneumonia. Pfizer immediately committed so much money into vaccine production on January 10, 2020. This fact came from Pfizer's own words in the *New England Journal of Medicine* article published on December 10, 2020. On January 14, 2020, four days after Pfizer went into vaccine production, the WHO Director General, Tedros Ghebreyesus, sent out a Tweet that there was no need to worry about Covid-19. Ten days later on January 24, 2020, despite all his knowledge about SARS-CoV-1, Dr. Anthony Fauci, an infectious disease expert and head of the US National Institute of Allergy and Infectious Diseases (NIAID), announced that there was no need for Americans to worry about Covid-19. Yet he knew about the Gain of Function GOF research. Dr. Fauci probably also knew about the genetically engineered coronavirus patented by the Pirbright Institute back in September 2014. The Pirbright Institute had applied for a coronavirus patent with the US Patent and Trademark Office on July 5, 2010. The brief description of the application was for

"A chimeric coronavirus S protein, with extended tissue tropism."

That's the same spike protein for which the mRNA vaccines were developed. The patent (#8828407) for this virus was granted on September 9, 2014 to three Pirbright inventors, Paul Britton, Erica Bickerton and Maria Arnesto. Exactly five weeks later, a three-page document was sent to different virology labs sponsored by the United States Government around the globe. The front page of this document, dated October 17, 2014 is shown on the next page. I found it while rummaging through Google for answers early in 2020. Dr. Fauci must have known about the Pirbright Institute's progress in developing a deadlier coronavirus. Of all the people that could be excused for not knowing the science of the SARS-CoV-2 virus, it isn't going to be Dr. Fauci.

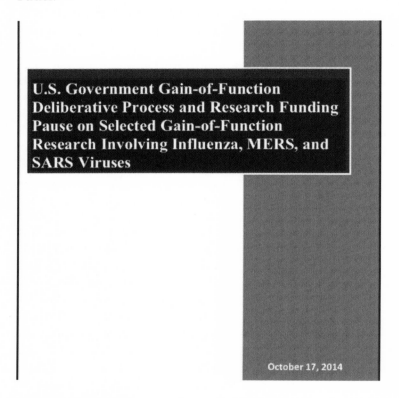

U.S. Government Gain-of-Function Deliberative Process and Research Funding Pause on Selected Gain-of-Function Research Involving Influenza, MERS, and SARS Viruses

October 17, 2014

On November 17, 2014, Jocelyn Kaiser posted a screen shot of the NIAID letter about halting gain-of-function testing. Dr. Fauci was fully aware of how contagious this virus was for years. He was trusted by nations not just by Americans. Many are still reeling from the negative impact of the misguided statements made by both Dr. Fauci and the WHO Director General. Virologists and healthcare professionals globally have been shocked by the un-curtailed nature of this current pandemic, with its politicization, polarization, profiteering, hidden secrets, overall poor management and misinformation. The knowledge gained from our experience with SARS-CoV-1 ought to have sufficed in handling the current pandemic. The global community was however misled and misinformed about the outbreak from the outset. According to Yale Professor of Pediatrics and Epidemiology, Warren Andiman, MD, the way the deadly Ebola outbreak in 2014-2015 as well as the 2003 SARS-CoV-1 outbreak were managed, shows we don't need any questionable high tech interventions to curtail Covid-19. In his 2018 book *Animal Viruses and Humans: A Narrow Divide*, Professor Andiman stated clearly that in response to SARS-CoV-1,

> *"Effectively, infection control and quarantine brought the disease to a halt in all the affected hotspots around the world." (Animal Viruses and Humans, p 119)*

Why aren't people around the world asking why the WHO misled or misinformed the entire world in January 14, 2020 on SARS-CoV-2? This blunder alone had a significant impact on the spread of the virus. Couple this to Dr. Fauci's misleading January 24, 2020 statement that there was nothing to be worried about despite his knowledge that the new virus SARS-CoV-2 was deadlier than SARS-CoV-1. You only need two such blunders to create a pandemic and there we have it. Contrast this with South Vietnam's success in curtailing the spread at the beginning of the pandemic.

The issue about blacklisting hydroxychloroquine or other treatments for Covid-19 has been resolved has been resolved in previous chapters and my book *The HCQ Debate*. A few puzzles still remain unsolved and one of these involves Pfizer's CEO. On November 9, 2020, Albert Bourla, the CEO of Pfizer, the world's first producer of the mRNA vaccine for Covid-19, sold 62% of his stock. There is nothing unusual about this day except it's the same day the US government ordered 300 million doses of Pfizer's mRNA vaccine. Some have informed me that this was merely a prudent business decision, and not Bourla's lack of confidence in his company's vaccine. I respect that but anything is possible. That's however not the only puzzle with Pfizer.

As of March 4, 2021, Mr. Bourla had not yet received the mRNA Covid vaccine. This would have gone unnoticed by the rest of the world except that he was denied entry into Israel because he was not yet vaccinated for Covid-19. A few proponents have shared their thoughts on this delayed vaccine and some have really good explanations as to why he hadn't received the vaccine three months after it was rolled out. You ought to watch Mr. Bourla's interview with CNN's Dr. Sanjay Gupta as well as the one with CNBC in December 2020. He claimed he and his family would take the vaccine once the "FDA approves it". Approved? Who can blame him! It's important to note Mr. Bourla's use of the word "approved" from a pharmaceutical company CEO regarding a drug. "Approved" is not the same as "authorized". What we have at the time of writing this second edition are "authorized" mRNA vaccines for Covid-19 not "approved" mRNA vaccines. That may soon change but Mr. Bourla is not interested in getting the vaccine just yet, while it is still in the "authorized" phase. I don't blame him. Do you? Getting "approval" requires filing an application with the FDA based on additional SAFETY and EFFICACY data. The CEO of a giant pharmaceutical company like Pfizer says he and his family would take the vaccine when it is "approved" by the FDA. It probably means he is not yet comfortable with the vaccine that only has FDA's "emergency use authorization" and not FDA approval. Your job on the other hand may mandate that you get the "authorized" not yet "approved" mRNA vaccine.

There may now be multiple commercial products on the market to help disrupt the transmission or progression of infection of SARS-CoV-2. This book is not intended to outline such products. I tried to reach the manufacturer of a new nasal spray but no one could get back with me in reasonable time. This wraps up the few remedies. Most of them have a scientific basis for helping you fight the invisible battle going on in your body.

Think clearly about your health and how you can improve it. Perhaps join a consumer advocate where there are both treating physicians and trusted scientists sharing information with the lay population in a safe respectful manner. You can also join Clubhouse® by downloading the app and looking for Covid-19 clubs discussing both early treatment, lies, liars, and the truth about all things Covid-19. That would help you gain a broader perspective and end most of the misinformation. It may also help you understand the human rights violations associated with the misinformation about vaccines and early treatment of Covid-19.

When you find health information, ask yourself if it is intentionally provided to make you believe there are no other effective treatments besides vaccines. I recently spoke to a doctor in charge of over 10,000 doctors around the world taking care of Covid-19 infected patients. He works with the WHO. He was very clear that early treatment is one of the reasons for their group's high success rate of over 99%. All the doctors in the group were also using safe, inexpensive, well-known drugs that have been around for a very long time. These are drugs the FDA has refused to acknowledge for treating Covid-19 here in the United States for whatever reason. That's partly why I had to write this book.

If something 'MAY WORK" in Covid-19 and if there are no other options, it ought to be used if it is indicated, it is safe and inexpensive, especially if it is recommended by a physician knowledgeable about and directly treating Covid-19 patients. It would be unethical to lie that such agents are ineffective and a crime against humanity to ensure that the information does not reach those that need it. Vaccines may be helpful, but you should not be coerced into getting vaccinated if you have concerns about its safety and efficacy and there are viable alternatives. The truth will eventually be revealed to us all about the extent of the vaccine's safety. That's my desire and prayer for now. With SARS-CoV-2, there are excellent alternatives suppressed by those who stand to gain the most from the pandemic.

If you're infected with Covid-19 or a long hauler of Covid-19, you should visit www.flccc.net as well as www.covidlonghaulers.com for more information and possibly help.

Chapter 22

The Book Amazon Blocked!

Could this book have helped lower infection and hospitalization rates if it had not been blocked on a popular publishing platform like Amazon? I think it would have. Amazon blocked it on April 8, 2020 under the guise of a flimsy excuse that "they" said not to publish the book. Till today, I don't know who "they" are. I had to find an IT person to make it available on my website for free. I'm sure you won't be surprised this happened by the time you've read this far. The only question I have is who are "they"? Do you know?

Many that downloaded the free book have shared it with others around the world. Thousands have been able to get the book from friends without any problems and I'm glad I kept it as a downloadable pdf document for easy sharing. Unlike the infomercials that take you to a website where you read a pdf-looking document that then disappears once you leave the page or your phone locks, the first edition of COVID-19 REMEDIES was still available offline to you after you left my website. Sharing the book with as many people as you wanted without having to go back to my website was important. I never placed an ad and anyone could download the free copy. The testimonials have been kept confidential because of the way Covid-19 has been politicized and abused. Clinic owners, healthcare professionals and others outside the healthcare profession have shared their gratitude with me. That included the awesome Governor of the state of Texas, Governor Gregg Abbott. Below is the picture of my author's page with Amazon's "BLOCKED".

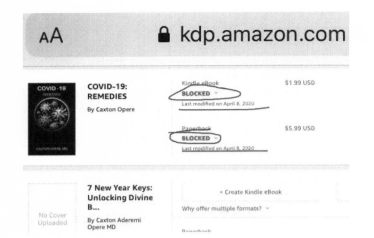

Strange as it might sound, even though Amazon blocked my book, they had published another Covid-19 book written by the Chinese Communist Party (CCP) at the same time. This book by the CCP on Covid-19 titled *Scheme for Diagnosis and Treatment of 2019 Novel Coronavirus Pneumonia* was on already on Amazon on April 8, 2020. The author listed on the front cover on the bottom left side of the book was the National Health Commission of the People's Republic of China. It had a nice light sky blue cover with a surgical mask at the center of the front cover. Here's the synopsis of my conversation with Amazon after I saw they had blocked the book you now have in your hands in its second edition:

> *Day 1, Wednesday April 8, 2020*
> *CSR = Customer Service Rep*
> ***Dr. Caxton**: Hi. Why did you block my book? We have a crisis that may eventually lead to the unnecessary deaths of so many people if the books contents are not made available. I'm not a taxicab driver whose grandmother just survived and now looking for 15 minutes of fame. This is ridiculous? This book is written to save lives!*

Amazon CSR: So sorry to hear that. Let's confirm your account. (Asks questions, clicks keyboard)

Dr. Caxton: Here it is. This is my 13ᵗʰ published book. We have a pandemic killing people and you block my book. Did you even read the book before blocking the book? I'm really disappointed.

Amazon CSR: *So sorry again. I see the book was blocked. No I didn't read the book. I am not one of the reviewers. I will find out what happened. Can you give me 24 hours? I will talk to the reviewers and call you back tomorrow morning.*

Dr. Caxton: *That would be fine.*

Day 2, Thursday April 9, 2020:

Amazon CSR: *(phone ringing). Hi. Is this Caxton Opere?*

Dr. Caxton: *Yes it is.*

Amazon CSR: *I spoke with the reviewers and they said "they" said not to publish the book.*

Dr. Caxton: *Who is "they"?*

Amazon CSR: *The reviewers said "They" said not to publish the book.*

Dr. Caxton: *This is crazy. A book like this during a pandemic should not be published? This is madness? You'd rather people die! What policy change allows you to block this book at a time like this?*

Amazon CSR: *Well, I will suggest you look at the published guidelines.*

Dr. Caxton: I have (Checks Amazon publishing guidelines again while on the phone with CSR). There's nothing here that says you can't publish the book. If anything, the guidelines make it clear you will publish my book even if there are dissenting views to what I have to say.

Amazon CSR: Since they said not to publish your book that's all I can say, I'm really sorry, Mr. Caxton.

Dr. Caxton: You're violating my right to free speech and endangering the American people at the same time. This is insanity! A disgrace. You're intentionally holding back information that can help Americans avoid large numbers of deaths during this pandemic. Unbelievable!

Amazon CSR: Sorry again but that's the policy.

Dr. Caxton: You will publish a book on the pandemic written by the Chinese Communist Party but refuse to publish my book? Then I will publish the book with or without Amazon.

Right after the phone conversation that Thursday morning, I called an IT expert to find out if he could put the book on my website. He said it could take up to three days. I told him to go ahead and also make the book free at www.doctorcaxton.com. On Saturday April 11, at 4:59pm, the IT guy called to say the book was now live and downloadable on the website. All visitors had to do was scroll down, enter their email and name once prompted and hit "subscribe". The pdf book would be sent to their email automatically. Some doctors and others called to say they tried to download the book 5 or six times and the site finally blocked them! They did not realize that the book had been emailed to them and thought it would be downloaded.

No one in their right mind would block a book like this from the American people. Doing so means they know what the book could do to stem the tide of expected deaths. Why would anyone block a book like this? It is simple, and contains helpful information to stem the tide of Covid-19 in the United States. Whoever does this had to be anti-American. I have upgraded the second edition to include more information I added several more remedies and of course famotidine and cetirizine.

What happened next, less than forty-eight hours after the book was released on my website, was a strange coincidence. It wasn't any different from the coincidence of Bill & Melinda Gates Foundation giving the Pirbright Institute $5.5 million in November 2019. The Bill and Melinda Gates Foundation had given the Pirbright Institute two other grants anything over $387,000 in grants prior to this date.

Stop Calling Herods Heroes!

Chapter 23

Cable Guy Break-in?

At about noon on Monday April 12, 2020, less than forty-eight hours after *Covid-19 Remedies* was available free on my website, my doorbell rang. My wife opened the door and a tall wiry guy without any protective gear saying he was from the cable company. He stood at the door requesting to enter the house. My wife told him we never called the cable company and didn't need his service. He insisted that we had called to schedule the appointment and that our neighbors had also complained about about poor Internet and cable reception. That wouldn't have been a problem except that we never called the cable company the entire weekend. My wife told him we never requested any service or reported any interruptions in Internet or cable service. By this time in the pandemic in 2020, most utility and service companies had trained or informed their staff to enter homes only with proper protective gear. No service personnel would come into your house without a facemask and gloves, perhaps with goggles or face shields in most states. My wife told him to wait, came to my study to inform me of this strange guy by the door insisting on getting into the house without any reason or an appointment. I put on a facemask, walked to the door and asked him again why he was here. Here's how the conversation went:

> **Dr. Caxton**: *How can I help you?*
>
> **Cable Guy**: *You guys called that you had a problem with your cable and I want to get in the house to see what the problem is.*
>
> **Dr. Caxton**: *I didn't call and neither did my wife.*

> *Cable Guy: You guys did call. I need to get in and see what's going on.*
>
> *Dr. Caxton: We did not call you and you are not coming inside. You see those cable boxes out there, you have my permission to do whatever you want there. But don't come near this house again. Good day.*

I was just inches away from the door outside with him. I stepped back in, told my wife this doesn't make any sense, and that if her phone rang in the next twenty seconds it means something strange was probably going on. That's exactly what happened. Her phone rang less than twenty seconds later! Though I don't know how they train their staff, the persistent eagerness this guy displayed, trying very hard to get into the house despite us telling him we didn't have an appointment, seemed completely out of place. If he was ringing a doorbell and they opened it and told him the cable or Internet reception was not having any problems, he shouldn't be trying to get in. Would you? It made no sense, particularly with Covid-19. He should be calling the dispatchers or whoever sent him to the house. Instead, he was so sure there was a problem inside our house he was trying to get in. I figured the guy was trying to enter my house for something suspicious. Yes, he came in the cable company vehicle.

Sensing something wasn't right about the guy, and the entire scenario, I told him "good day". If you are a spiritual individual you will understand what I mean when I say my spiritual antenna went on alert as it did at that moment. That's when I told my wife if her phone rang in the next twenty seconds, something fishy was going on. Why? It would take at least a minute for the cable guy to call his company dispatcher and explaining what went on in front of my door. Whoever the cable maintenance guy had called after I shut the door would also have had to make a few notes on a computer that was related to any file they had on us as their customer, unless they already had our file open before the guy called by coincidence. So unless he was streaming the entire interaction live while the conversation was going on in front of my door, which would be illegal without my permission, there was no way my wife's phone should be ringing in less than twenty seconds after I closed the door.

Nevertheless, after I shut the door behind me and my wife's phone rang, she picked the call. It was a lady from the cable company. My wife told the caller to "hold on a second" as she brought the phone to me in my study. I was working on *COVID-19: Physician Treatment Strategies*, my second book on Covid-19. The caller wanted to know why we sent the guy away.

Here's how that conversation went:

> *Cable Lady: Hi. You guys called that you were having problems with your cable*
>
> *Dr. Caxton: No we didn't. You must have the wrong address.*
>
> *Cable Lady: (States my address correctly). Is this your address?*
>
> *Dr. Caxton: Yes, but we never called you.*
>
> *Cable Lady: Sure you did. You called sometime over the weekend.*
>
> *Dr. Caxton: Let me ask you something. This is becoming ridiculous. When exactly over the weekend did we call you guys to make the appointment?*

> **Cable Lady**: *I'm not sure but I know it was sometime over the weekend.*
>
> **Dr. Caxton**: *Really? Can you tell me exactly what day it was? Friday, Saturday or Sunday?*
>
> **Cable Lady**: *No I can't, but I'm sure you did call. Several neighbors also called about interruption to their Internet and cable service.*
>
> **Dr. Caxton**: *Let's cut to the chase here. You want to enter my house based on a request I didn't make and you're telling me I made the request. Yet you can't tell me which day or time I called the cable company. Are you kidding me? Please don't call back and don't send anyone near my property again. The work I'm doing is one of national security and you'll need a high security clearance letter from the President of United States to get inside my house. Have a good day!*

My wife went out later that evening to ask at least four different neighbors if they had any interruptions to their Internet or cable over the weekend. Not too surprisingly, none of them had any such issues. The next day, Tuesday April 13, 2020 as I was driving to the emergency room, my wife called me. She told me there was a guy parked on the other side of the street in a cable company vehicle. He had been trying to convince her to let him in the house for more than five minutes and she had told him no. He tried to be as pleasant as possible and for just one goal, getting into the house. I contacted a friend who recommended security measures. That wasn't all that happened but I'll leave the rest to your imagination.

Chapter 24

You Should Never Give Up!

As you come to the end of the book, I want you to think about your life goals. I would like to share some tools with you in the form of questions to stir you up or put you back on track on your life's journey. I hope to put some desire, energy and fire in you and inspire you to greatness with these questions.

First, why are you here on earth?" Everyone was born into this world with a purpose. Asking this question and taking whatever steps necessary to answer it will expose you to limitless possibilities. No matter what you've lost or continue to lose as a result of Covid-19, you must know why you are here, your real purpose. Not what your parents, teachers, uncles, aunts, principals, professors, employers or spouses want from you. These people were necessary for you to begin developing a sense of identity, a set of rules for living, a sense of purpose, and may be a significant source of continuous encouragement, love and support. Nevertheless, there comes a time when you have to severe ties with them mentally, emotionally and perhaps physically and financially, if you are going to discover who you really are. The only person that should remain in your field of vision is your spouse and your children if you have any.

Therefore shall a man leave his father and his mother, and shall cleave unto his wife: and they shall be one flesh. Genesis 2:26.

These individuals, no matter how much they love you, may stand in your way of identifying and fulfilling your true calling on planet earth. You'll need to leave these individuals at least metaphorically as a mature adult in order to develop clarity, a sense of identity, a very firm grip on yourself, and be able to pursue your true purpose. It doesn't matter what you've lost or don't have. What matters is that you're here right now! Find a way through books, coaches, courses, friends, groups online learning. Joining groups of like-minded achievers who have done what you're hoping to accomplish or better will polish your gifts and present you with greater opportunities. They'll help you see what chasms lie between where you are now and where you need to be and what to expect along the way. Never ever give up. The world needs you, pain, losses, and all.

The world needs you, pain, losses, and all! We need you!

You can't imagine how much your pain can help another see that there is hope until you try. If you're feeling so down that you feel like giving up, I'm sure there's at least one person on this planet waiting to hear your story and be encouraged by it. Your story will help somebody trying to give up on life. I recommend you watch or listen to Les Brown's story *Choosing Your Future*. You'll be a different person by the time you're done with it. But you must promise that you will share story with other! This may be the thing for which you'll always be remembered. Your willingness to share your story could also be the one thing that completely changes your life for good. Remember, everything you dream of is possible, hard, dependent on you, worth it and can come to pass.

Secondly, what do you want to be remembered for? What battles do you want to be remembered for in the history books of winners? Maya Angelou said,

"You may not control all the events that happen to you but you can decide not to be reduced by them."

A lot has happened in the last seventeen months, most of it unquantifiable losses: bankruptcies, breakups, deaths, disappointments, divorce, foreclosures, and so much more pain. Yet some have been able to take all that pain and loss and turned it into gain. How were they able to do it and how are you going to be able to do it, even if you're still reeling in pain? It's by focusing on the answer to the first question, "why am I here?" I believe we only have two choices in life and therefore only two paths, mediocrity or greatness. There's no middle ground. You can only choose one or the other. It's either mediocrity or greatness. You do so consciously or unconsciously by your daily actions. If you're reading this book, I believe it's because you know about greatness and prefer it to mediocrity, you know about choices and you want to make the best ones. You're one of that rare breed of humans on the planet who will not take no for an answer. Even when doctors can't tell you what to do, you're seeking for answers on your own. That's the trait common to those who downloaded the first edition of this book. If you're reading this far, you've got something special in you. Don't let it die unannounced, unused, unappreciated, or uncelebrated. Don't give up on your dreams no matter how hard the demands for their fulfillment. Make a down payment using the most valuable currency in the world, your words.

For by thy words thou shalt be justified, and by thy words thou shalt be condemned. Matthew 12:27

The third question is, what is the secret sauce you need to help you fulfill your purpose? In order to answer this third question, I'll introduce you to one of my heroes, Nick Vujicic. If you know Nick, skip this paragraph. Nick, born in December 1982, has the greatest smile in the world. He is happily married to the beautiful Kanae Miyahara and they have four children. He is also the best selling author of *Unstoppable* and several other books. So what's so special about Nick? In your mind Nick might be a 6-foot tall, athletic all American star. Wrong! Nick was born with no arms and no legs, that's what so special about Nick! He was born with what's called tetra-amelia. Today he is known all around the world for inspiring others. He shares how he wanted to commit suicide at a young age because of his congenital deficits. He now lifts up those around him to greater heights of purpose and power and shares how God became a major player in his life. If a man like Nick can find happiness, so can you. You need to find the secret source for your happiness, particularly during this tragic period of our human history of horrific losses. Nick's superpower is his attitude of gratitude. He is not going around with a sad look blaming God for tetra-amelia syndrome, he is grateful to be alive. As long as you can breathe, find a reason to be grateful.

Jessica Moore, one of my hungry to speak members in the Les Brown Family of Speakers was a single parent with no support. She wanted to go to college. To ease this journey, she decided she wanted to be a resident advisor. That would enable her get free rent and a good and flexible job. Against all odds, she volunteered at the college's housing department while still working as a cashier. She poured her soul into the students and helped transform their lives. In Jessica's own words,

"It got to a point where students would request my help but I didn't work there. Then one day, I received a call to the director's office. I'm thinking, what did I do? We met, and he said you have been transforming the lives of the students and you haven't even given yourself credit. The area coordinator then said…"Bring your direct deposit form so we can put you on payroll". I became the FIRST nontraditional resident advisor. …And just like that, I had a job that allowed me to continue school, bring my daughter with me and our rent, bills and food, were PAID for IN FULL."

I had an opportunity to interview Jessica and obtain her permission to share her story in this book. She agreed. I was also able to ask her wonderful daughter, 9-year old Raivyn, if she wanted to see her name mentioned in this book. Raivyn was of course delighted. She is now planning to be a motivational speaker!

Your loss may be great but your greatness lies ahead of you. Just don't give up, not now. Here's an anthem of for your soul,

> *Clear your mind of danger, death, debris, defeat, depression, destruction and disease. Define your purpose and dance in it. Rise in defiance against those disturbing elements with dogged determination and divine approval. Dare to be different. Do what you've never done before and life will give you what you've never had before. Charge forward with the call of destiny ringing in your heart with a renewed spirit that cannot be defeated. Never ever give up. If you won't stop you, nothing, no one else can stop you. Do it and dance to your own beat. Dance.*

No friends? Don't give up. No family? Don't give up. No job? Don't give up. No money? Don't give up. Lost everything? Don't give up. Down on your back? Then look up. For if you can look up, you can get up!

Testimonials have been removed to protect the identity of the wonderful people who have shared the knowledge and benefits they got from the first edition with their clients and families.

A portion of the sales from this book is donated to Frisco Family Services. The first edition of this book was a free downloaded shared with many others. Please support the work we do by ordering multiple copies of the book. Amazon kept the book blocked since April 8, 2020:

Kindly circulate the information and do all you can to stay safe and inform others. Tell your healthcare providers to get their own copies.

Drop your comments at
www.doctorcaxton.com
https:m.facebook.com/public/Caxton-Aderemi-Opere

About The Author

Dr. Caxton Opere is a board-certified internist, frontline Covid-19 physician who has worked with the US Covid-19 task force as a frontline critical care physician. He is the world's # 1 authority on the medical complications of divorce as well as the pioneer of the 5-Minute Compatibility Test. He has been a practicing Internal medicine, critical care and emergency medicine physician for over 31 years, and the former Medical Director of the HIV/AIDS Ryan White Program at Capitol City Family Health Center in Baton Rouge Louisiana. He received Tumblr's 2015 Award for 100 Best Startups for his Divorce Medicine Project, and was recognized by the Louisiana Senate for his work in Divorce Prevention and by Texas Governor Gregg Abbott for his books on treatment of Covid-19. He is an International Speaker and author of several books. As a relationship expert he helps divorced professionals remarry confidently. He has had the opportunity to meet with some of the most highly sought after celebrities and media personalities around the world including Dr. Phil, Les Brown, Kimora Lee, Dolph Lundgren, Gary Kasparov, Stedman Graham, retired psychiatrist, addiction expert and radio show host, Winn Henderson, MD. He also runs the weekly 3R Relationship Room on Clubhouse.

Made in the USA
Monee, IL
04 October 2021

79310084R00072